contents

get set

Kids want to be active. All the research confirms it. And it's up to us, as parents, to help our children to build more activity and fitness into their lives.

Greater activity will:

- improve your kids self-confidence
- give them more energy
- improve alertness and concentration
- help them to sleep at night
- keep them fit and trim.

Fostering a love of being active now will set them up for a fit and healthy future, and last them a lifetime.

But, activity does not have to mean sport or exercise. You and your child can reap the health benefits of doing more in all sorts of fun, simple and unusual ways – there are plenty of family-friendly and affordable activity suggestions in Chapter Three that will appeal to the sporty, the non-sporty and the plain lazy.

Naturally, the food your kids eat also plays a big part in their health profile, so there will be advice on how to eat the right foods without turning mealtimes into a battle.

You'll also find essential guidance on:

- motivating your child
- making more time for activity
- activities for non-sporty and overweight kids
- finding the right sport
- converting couch potatoes into fit kids
- identifying your child's fitness personality
- how to make it all fun.

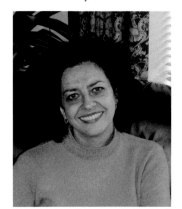

As the mother of two adolescent boys, I know the importance of finding the right activities to keep children keen and positively involved. Rest assured, however, that with a little imagination and the right sort of encouragement your children could be fit and healthy for life.

Claire Gillman

getting *your* kids active

how to
have active,
healthy kids

claire gillman

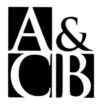

First published 2007 by

A & C Black Publishers Ltd
38 Soho Square, London W1D 3HB
www.acblack.com

Copyright © 2007

ISBN–10: 0 7136 8141 1
ISBN–13: 978 0 7136 8141 3

A CIP catalogue record for this book is available from the British Library.

Note: It is always the responsibility of the individual to assess his or her own fitness capability before participating in any training activity. Whilst every effort has been made to ensure the content of this book is as technically accurate as possible, neither the author nor the publishers can accept responsibility for any injury or loss sustained as a result of the use of this material.

Text and cover design by James Watson
Cover photograph © courtesy of Blend Images LLC/istockpro.com

The publishers would like to thank the following for permission to use photographs:
Silhouettes of kids in motion © Superstock (www.rubberball.com)
Kid's food © Bananastock
All other photos © www.istock.com

This book is produced using paper that is made from wood grown in managed, sustainable forests. It is natural, renewable and recyclable. The logging and manufacturing processes conform to the environmental regulations of the country of origin.

Typeset in Garamond by Fakenham Photosetting Limited
Printed and bound in China by WKT

acknowledgements

As ever, I'd like to thank my husband Nick, for his unswerving support – particularly as deadlines loomed; and to my two wonderful and boisterous sons, Alex and George, for giving me the inspiration for this book, and the opportunity to practice what I preach. I would also like to thank my literary agent and friend Chelsey Fox for her editorial wisdom, and thanks to Charlotte Croft at A&C Black for making the book possible.

dedication

To Sarah
I dedicate this book to my cousin, Sarah Penfold (née Edmonds: 8th December 1970–30th June 2006) who tragically died of cancer last year.

foreword

For the past 12 years I have worked with thousands of children who have been inactive and as a consequence have struggled with their weight. It is with great pleasure that I write the foreword for this book as I have witnessed firsthand the challenges children and their parents face in today's society, in trying to lead an active healthy lifestyle.

Physical activity levels are low in virtually every sector of our society. According to the most recent UK government statistics, approximately two-thirds of men, three-quarters of women and one-third of our children do not meet the levels needed to prevent the development of a broad range of chronic diseases. These figures reflect the many changes that have occured within our homes, schools, communities and work places, creating a more time- and energy-efficient society, which as a result promotes inactivity.

A book which can provide parents with simple, realistic and supportive information from an author who understands the challenges faced by parents in today's society is a welcome addition. This book is packed with useful facts, helpful tips and inspirational ideas which will help parents to make their children's lifestyle more active, enjoyable and healthy.

Peter Mackreth BA (Hons), PGCE, MSc.
Senior Lecturer in Physical Activity & Obesity Management
Leeds Metropolitan University

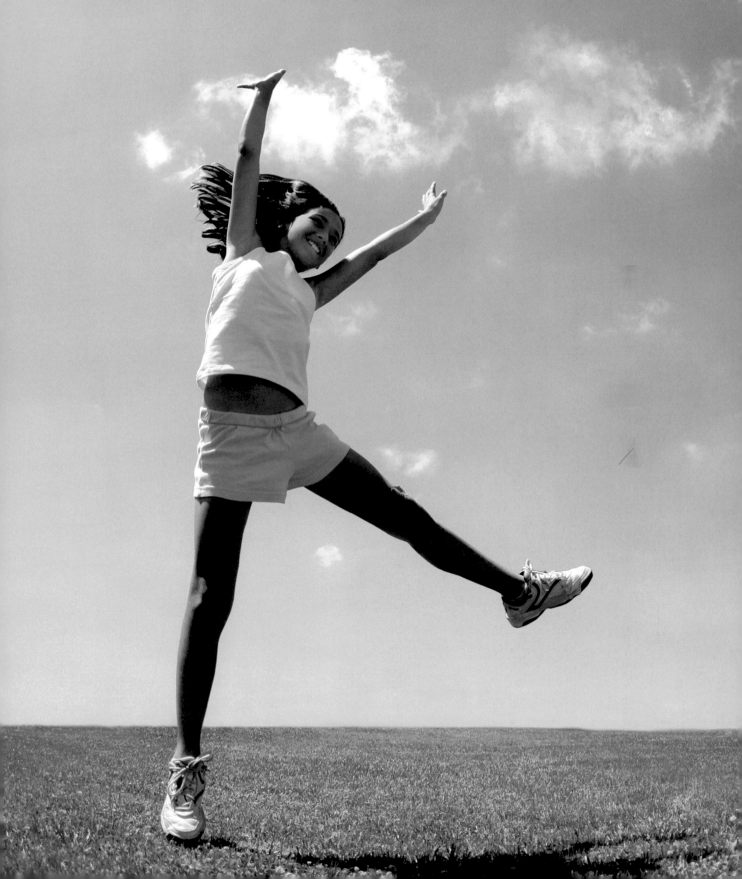

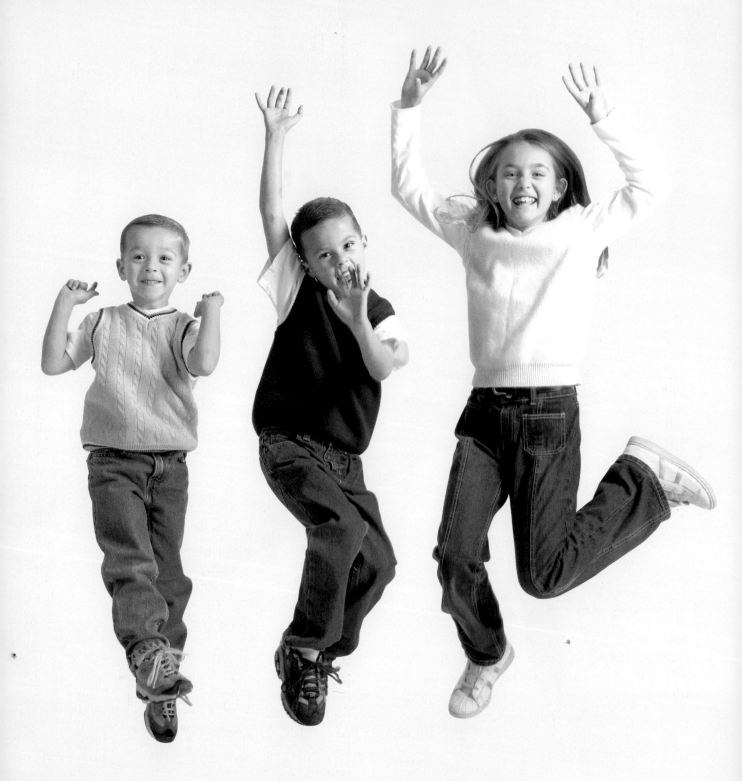

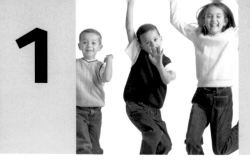

why act now?

The good news is that you are well placed to get your children active and eating healthily, albeit that it will take some dedication and probably a change in the way that your family approaches eating and exercise.

The bad news is that there is no time to lose. The statistics make pretty scary reading. Childhood obesity is at an all-time high and today's youth are playing less sport and are involved in less activity than ever before.

According to the National Audit Office, nearly one-third of children between the ages of 2 and 15 are overweight or obese. With today's sedentary lifestyles, more children than ever before are at risk of becoming overweight and suffering from the inherent health and emotional ramifications that entails.

The British Medical Association's *Preventing Childhood Obesity* report (June 2005) says that children who are obese have a much higher chance of suffering from illnesses such as:

- certain cancers – specifically breast and bowel cancer

- type II diabetes

- high blood pressure

- coronary heart disease

- arthritis

- sleep-related disorders

- menstrual problems

- increased risk of fractures, broken bones and joint pain.

Being overweight and out of shape can also have damaging psychological and painful emotional effects on children. This may lead to low self-esteem, low self-image and depression, and can be the cause of underachievement in later life.

fact *In the UK, the number of obese children has tripled in 20 years. One in ten six-year-olds is now obese. On present trends, half of all children in 2020 could be obese.*

So why are we in this mess?

With greater access to information and heightened public health awareness, how, you might ask, have we come to this? In fact it's a question that has also been vexing the experts, and there is little consensus on the answer. Generally, what is agreed is that lifestyle changes, such as greater use of cars and more sedentary jobs/leisure time, combined with dietary changes, such as the rise in convenience foods and snacking, are the major contributory factors. However, the problem is much more complex than it at first appears.

Parental fears

The media is keen to label the latest 'computer-game' generation as lazy. Yet, inadvertently, it is our generation who are contributing to our children's sedentary lifestyles.

Despite improvements in road, car and playground safety, studies show that parents today are more fearful for their children than they were 30 years ago. In most cases our fears are completely unfounded. For example, in 2004 the Department of Transport recorded that the number of children under the age of 15 killed either in cars or as pedestrians was 166 – that's a reduction of 75 per cent on the 1976 figure.

In spite of this evidence to the contrary, many parents (myself included) still worry that it is not safe for their children to walk to school alone, reasoning that there is so much more traffic and people drive so much faster than in our day. (Tips on getting your children to school can be found in Chapter Two.)

The other fear that haunts all parents is that of abduction or 'stranger danger'. Yet the number of child murders has remained more or less constant over the past 30 years. The sad truth is that the culture of fear that dominates modern-day parenting is restricting our children's independent outdoor lives.

Even though many of us are intuitively aware that these fears are ungrounded, no parent wants to take the risk with their own child's safety. It is this parental 'belts and braces' approach to protection that prevents kids today from enjoying the freedoms of the past to run, cycle and play at large, or simply to walk to school on their own.

WHAT IS OBESITY?

The Faculty of Public Health defines obesity as 'an excess of body fat frequently resulting in a significant impairment of health and longevity'. Clear as mud, isn't it, and even harder to apply. A more useful yardstick to obesity is to measure your child's Body Mass Index (BMI) (see charts on pages 111–12) or to consult your GP.

fact *In the Government's Time Life Survey 2000, it was found that two-thirds of the population do very little or no sporting activity.*

SWALLOWS AND AMAZONS

There are concerns that today's 'cotton-wool' generation are failing to learn the risk-taking skills necessary for adult life because of overprotective parents and schools.

In response, the government's children's commissioner Al Aynsley-Green intends to launch a campaign to encourage and help schools to restore more challenging physical extra-curricular activities such as adventure training expeditions, camping and walking trips.

Aynsley-Green, a former professor of child health at Great Ormond Street Hospital, cites organisations such as the Scouts, Girl Guides, the Duke of Edinburgh's Award and the Outward Bound Trust as those that offer the chance for children to learn about physical risk.

fact *In 1971, eight out of ten eight-year-olds walked to school alone. Now it is less than one in ten. Back then, by the age of 11 almost every child used to walk, but the number now has tumbled to 55 per cent and is still falling.*

High pressure living

Safety is not the only reason for parents' caution. Practicality and logistics also fuel the trend to drive our children everywhere. The noblest intentions of walking with the children to school can be thwarted by the reality that, owing to the pressures of modern living, many parents drop their children by car en route to work or some other commitment. (See Chapter Two for ways to get round this problem.)

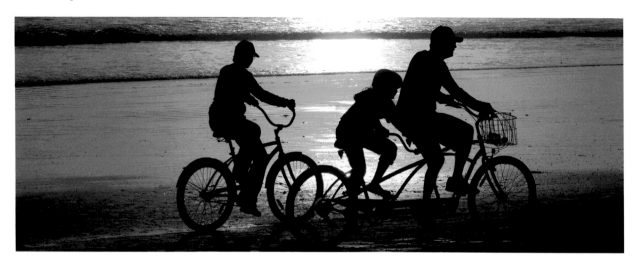

STARTLING CAR STATISTICS

- The proportion of primary-school children being driven to school has increased by one-third over the past decade, from 30 per cent to 41 per cent.

- Four in ten children are taken to school by car, compared to less than one in ten in 1971.

- Only one in twenty children use their bicycles for transport in the UK. Car travel accounts for 80 per cent of the total distance travelled by the UK population.

- There are some 30 million vehicles in the UK.

Bad food choices

High-fat, high-calorie foods, commonly described as 'energy dense' because they are highly calorific without being correspondingly filling, have become a staple of the British diet. And it is a simple truth that if a child consumes more calories than he burns he will become overweight.

There are other factors that also affect the likelihood of a child piling on the pounds – body type, home life, activity levels etc. – but even if your child can eat junk food like there's no tomorrow and still look like a string bean, this kind of diet will be damaging his physical well-being and storing up health problems for the future.

So why are children overeating?

- Grazing and snacking rather than eating regular main meals has become the norm.

- Until recent initiatives, such as the Jamie Oliver's School Dinners campaign, food and drink provided in schools has been heavy in fat, salt and sugar.

- Many schools now provide vending machines for students.

■ Families no longer eat together. It has become commonplace for family members to grab food to fit in with their schedules and many children and adults eat in front of the television or 'on the run'.

■ Portion sizes have grown substantially in the last 20 years. As a result, many families are out of touch with what constitutes a normal portion.

■ Food manufacturers target children and influence their food preferences with clever advertising and marketing campaigns.

MEALS ON THE GO

By 2009, it is estimated that Brits will consume nearly 3 billion less main meals at home, with breakfast being the most frequently missed meal. In addition, eating 'on the go' is on the up for 2006 – British consumers spent around £8 billion on food while on the move, representing an average of £170 per person a year.

'Some kids are getting up to 40 per cent of their total calorific value from snack foods and we just don't know what the combined effects of this are. We have no idea what it's doing to their health.'

Dr Martin Caraher, Reader in Food & Health Policy at City University.

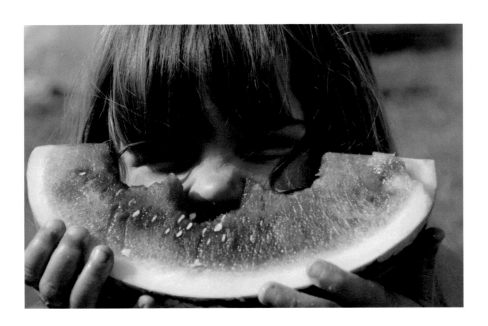

Food temptations

For all of us, food is inextricably linked with our emotions. If you understand the role food plays in your household you can better understand why some children struggle to resist overeating.

- **Food as love**: From the moment our babies are placed in our arms we sustain and nurture them and show our love for them with food. The toddler who falls and grazes his knee is given a sweet to 'make it better'. Sometimes we pop a child's favourite treat into his lunchbox to remind him that we're thinking of him. It is small wonder then that in the minds of our children food is love. And the withdrawal of food is the withdrawal of love.

- **Food as reward**: If your child does well at school, very often he will receive some kind of sugary treat. The reward for a good report or good SAT results is perhaps a meal out.

- **Food as celebration**: Birthdays and holidays such as Christmas and Easter are marked by a celebratory cake or meal. The more important the occasion the more lavish the food.

- **Food as pleasure**: Let's face it, food tastes great and it can be enormously pleasurable. Unfortunately, for many kids, it is the high-fat, salty and sugary foods that are most irresistible.

- **Food is sociable**: We join our friends for dinner and relax over a meal out. Naturally, our children follow suit and, as they become more independent (and before alcohol takes on a role in their lives), meeting for a burger or fried chicken becomes part of their social structure, and an expectation after outings to the cinema etc.

- **Food as power**: Children are quick to learn that food provides them with power. From the faddy eater who gets massive amounts of attention to the sibling who seeks praise and approval by 'clearing his plate', there are huge opportunities for manipulating parents.

fact *Your child only needs to exceed his calorie needs by one can of fizzy drink per day to pile on 7 kg (15 lb) in a year.*

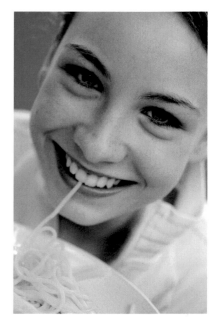

Finding a solution

Should we blame the exploding obesity epidemic on gluttony, sloth or both? Well, in the UK, the Health Select Committee's report of 2004 was clear: 'It is crucial that both sides of the "energy equation" are addressed', it stated. That means finding ways to reduce people's intake of food – especially certain types of food – while encouraging them to exercise more.

The report notes that:

- The average person now walks 304 km (189 miles) per year compared to 410 km (255 miles) 20 years ago.

- Levels of cycling have fallen by more than 80 per cent in the last 50 years.

- Less than 1 per cent of school journeys are now made by bicycle.

- Half the nation's children fail to achieve the government's target of two hours activity per week.

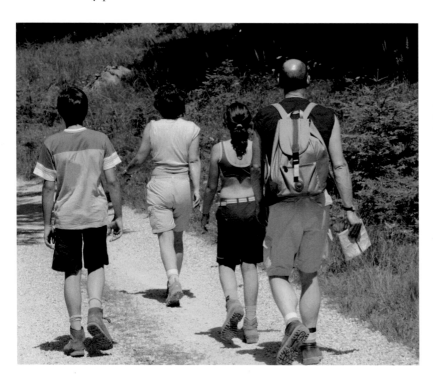

fact *For the first time in recent history, it is believed that life expectancy for this generation of overweight or obese children will be shorter than that of their parents.*

CHILDHOOD OBESITY

The 2002 Health Survey for England noted that more than one in five boys and more than one in four girls were either overweight or obese. If you project these figures forwards by 15 years, simply by assuming a steady growth, it suggests that around one-third of adults will be obese by 2020. However, **'if the rapid acceleration in childhood obesity in the last decade is taken into account, the predicted prevalence in children for 2020 will be in excess of 50 per cent.'**

(*RCP, Storing up problems*)

At the same time, energy-dense foods are becoming increasingly available. Paradoxically, calorie consumption per capita has fallen by 20 per cent since 1970. Nonetheless, the Royal College of General Practitioners points out that, although food intake has fallen on average by 750 kcal per day, activity levels have fallen by 800 kcal. Crucially, the wave of obesity has come out of this small imbalance.

The Committee's report concludes:

'It is clear that people are overeating in relation to their energy needs, and that the cheapness, availability and heavy marketing of energy-dense foods makes this very easy to do, coupled with an increasing reliance on snacks and ready-prepared meals which makes selecting "healthy" foods harder.'

Official dithering

Somewhat ironically, given the Select Committee findings, the final factor that contributes to our children's ever-expanding waistlines may well be red tape and officialdom.

An influential report published in February 2006 by three government watchdogs concluded that red tape and a lack of leadership are jeopardising efforts to tackle Britain's growing childhood obesity crisis.

It took 31 experts 18 months merely to agree how obesity should be measured. This delay means it is likely to be 2007 before children are routinely weighed and measured.

The report identified that:

- The numerous government departments, quangos and local bodies, such as teachers and healthcare professionals, responsible for implementing obesity strategy were unclear about their roles.

- There are insufficient front-line staff with the right skills.

- There are countless 'initiatives' but no specific money to implement them.

- There is, as yet, no clear evidence or agreement of which strategies will work.

FOOD ADVERTISING TO CHILDREN

In July 2004, the government's Food Standards Agency (FSA) reported that a systematic review of the link between food promotion and children's eating behaviour had found that TV advertising of sugared breakfast cereals, soft drinks, confectionery and savoury snacks, closely followed by fast-food outlets, affects the preferences of children and what they buy or pester parents to buy.

The FSA agreed that action was required on the promotion of foods that are high in fat, sugar and salt if the balance of children's diets is to be improved. In 2007, adverts for these products during programmes for children under sixteen were banned.

While recognising that it is difficult to try to change established habits in schools and in society generally, the overriding message of the report is that confusion, lack of leadership, shortage of evidence and lack of accountability means that our children grow fatter while the experts and the 'delivery chain' dithers.

What can be done?

Although the facts make fairly grim reading, there is a great deal about which to be positive. As I said in the introduction, not only is it possible with a little determination to get your children on the move and eating more healthily, but it can also be great fun. Moreover, the time and effort that you invest now will be more than repaid in the future by your children's good health and fitness.

In this book, I wish to show ways to:

- build more activity into your daily lives

- eat more healthily

- instil positive fitness and eating habits that will last a lifetime.

To achieve these goals, we broadly follow these basic principles:

- making it fun and imaginative

- doing it as a family

- making healthy eating and activity as accessible as possible.

US researchers suggest that obesity risks could be cut by around one-third if the average TV viewing time decreased from 3 hours a day to 1 hour a day. Currently, most overweight children watch more than 3 hours per day and about 25 per cent of all US high-school students watch more than 4 hours per day. In the UK, the average for secondary-school students is somewhat lower at between 2 and 3 hours per day.

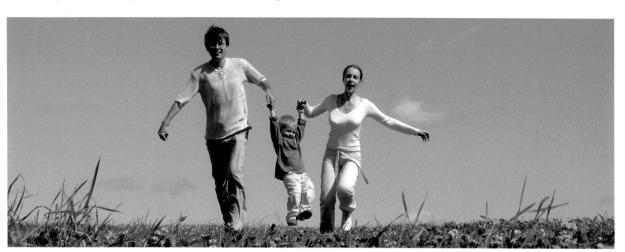

If kids eat well, why do they need exercise?

Diet obviously plays an important part in making sure kids remain healthy and do not pile on the pounds, but the other essential part of the equation is for kids to be more active. Exercise is vital for children to build healthy bones and muscles, and it helps them sleep better at night and remain more alert during the day. But the benefits extend far beyond keeping fit and trim.

MORE GOOD NEWS

Kids who play sport develop better nutritional habits for life, according to a study in the *Journal of the American Dietetic Association*. Researchers at the University of Minnesota questioned nearly 5000 teenagers and found that the active ones ate breakfast, dinner and healthy snacks more often than the others. Even those who took part in sports such as distance running and gymnastics, where there is pressure to stay lean, showed better eating habits.

Activity:

- improves their self-confidence,
- teaches important lessons about teamwork and losing with good grace
- gives more energy for every aspect of their lives,
- produces better performance in the classroom.

Team spirit

The best way to get your child more active is to get the whole family involved. Parents and kids alike need to work together as a team to achieve good health and well-being. That means:

- **Being active together**: Making it usual for the family to be active, not sedentary.
- **Eating together**: Eating a healthy meal together as a family is great for socialising, inspiring your child to try new foods and reinforcing the messages about good nutrition.

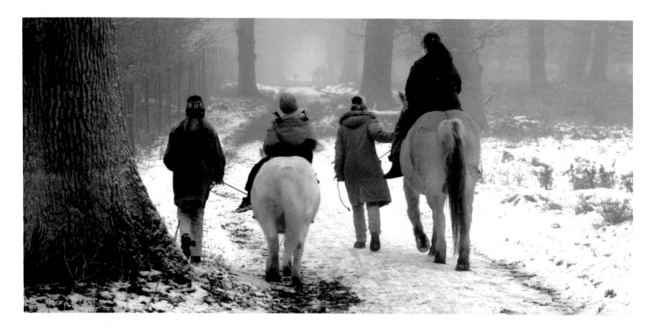

- **Being a role model**: As in any team, there is a leader and it is part of your role to set the kind of example that you know your kids need.

- **Laying the foundation**: By encouraging healthy habits now, you will enable your child to make wise choices as he becomes more independent.

OFFICIAL SUPPORT

Although your parental role is pivotal in getting your child to be more active, all elements of society – from government to industry to schools – bear some responsibility for making improvements in the way we collectively approach healthy living. The good news is that the message is starting to get through. The government is investing in some exciting new community sports opportunities that are available for everyone and, with the advent of a greater number of television channels, less conventional sports and activities are starting to get airtime to inspire our children.

(For more information on local and government initiatives, see Chapter Four and for 'alternative activities' turn to Chapter Three.)

fact *London hosting the Olympics in 2012 has fired up children's enthusiasm. A Norwich Union survey in August 2005 showed that almost half said they would love to represent Britain in 2012 and nearly one-third intend to increase the amount of sport and exercise they do in a bid to get chosen for the Games.*

How to use this book

Soon, you'll be armed with all the information and advice that you need to start making positive changes in your family's daily life. As you'll see, these changes do not have to be dramatic. In fact, the overriding message is to take small, subtle steps towards a more active lifestyle, so that these simple changes become an integral part of life and are easier to maintain.

This book does not offer a prescriptive programme to follow. Rather, it is a collection of ideas that will help you to adopt the principles of being active and eating right into your own family situation.

It is written and designed in such a way that you can read it in one go, or you can dip in and out – seeking out the relevant chapter for the particular scenario that you are facing. Perhaps your child eats relatively well, but has no inclination to abandon his 'couch-potato' lifestyle. In which case, the section on motivation is more relevant to you than the section on dealing with faddy diets, for example.

Depending on how entrenched your child is in his sedentary ways, your moves towards a healthier lifestyle may be challenging. However, given that the growing tide of overweight children and adults shows no sign of abating, making positive changes towards a more active lifestyle now is a lifelong gift for you to give to your children.

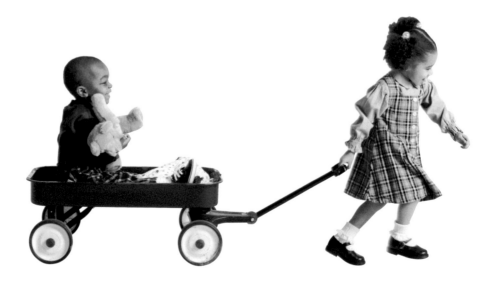

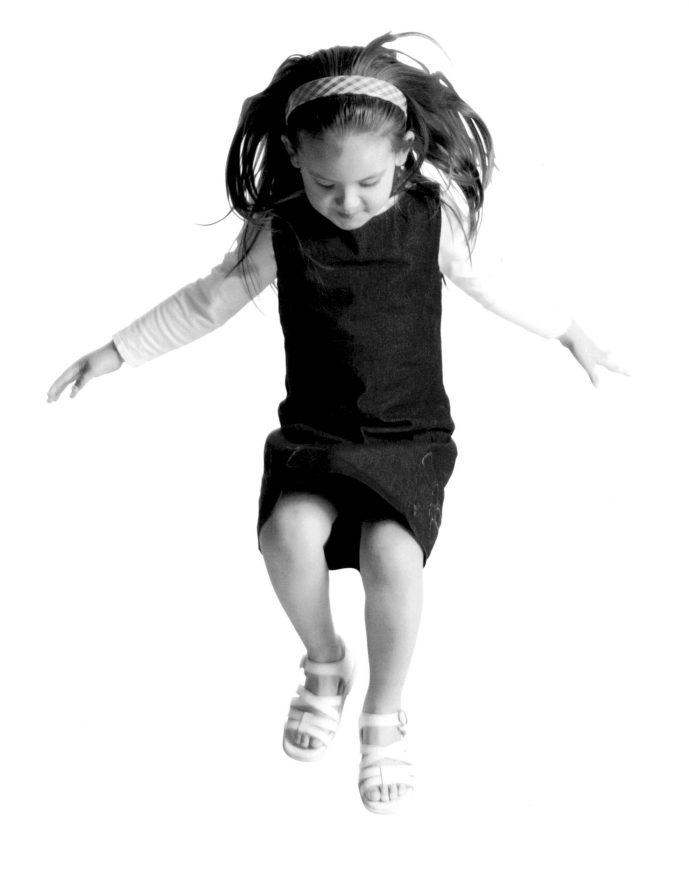

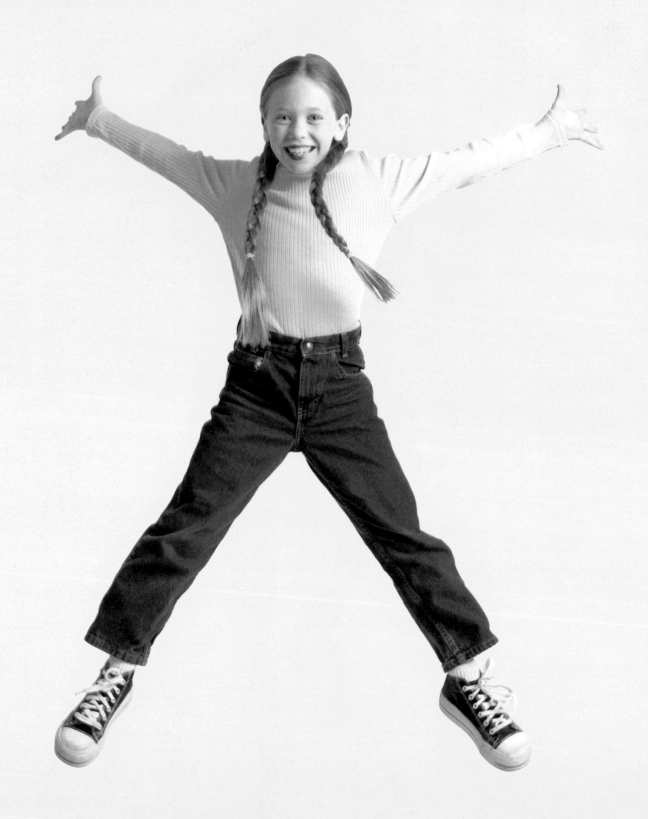

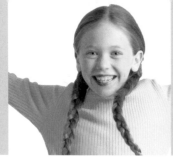

2 developing a positive approach

It is unreasonable to expect children to take responsibility for their own fitness. Also, with schools required to offer only two hours of organized physical activity a week (and many not even able to deliver this), you cannot count on your child's education to provide a positive foundation on which to build.

Realistically, to foster a positive approach to activity in your child will require a team effort involving the whole family – with you as the main instigator! It needs you to be upbeat and positive about activity rather than a nag or passive observer. Activity has to be seen as fun and as an integral part of daily life rather than as a chore.

Formula for happiness

How do you make something that is anathema to your unfit child appear fun? Well, firstly, you must believe it yourself. So, here's the theory to back up your arguments.

When Prof. Michael Argyle was Emeritus Professor of Psychology at Oxford Brookes University in the 1990s he studied what constitutes happiness (or 'subjective well-being' as it's known in scientific circles). He discovered that there are certain key factors which are present in many physical activities that help our kids to be happy and to enjoy their sport. These vital factors are:

■ **Natural highs:** Exercise produces a positive mood because of the release of endorphins (the body's natural 'uppers') into the bloodstream. Combine this with the rush of adrenalin produced by high-excitement activities or competitive sports and, physiologically, your child is well on the way to feeling happy.

■ **Go with the flow**: When your child starts to master the necessary skill to perform an activity well, and it all comes together, then she is experiencing what is known as 'flow'. Professor Argyle once said, 'When a high level of challenge is met by a high level of skill, you get a deep sense of satisfaction known as flow. It's a loss of awareness, brought about by facing challenges with necessary skills.' Prof. Argyle put a lot of emphasis on the skill factor in achieving happiness. He believed that enjoying your skill – and being noticed by others because of it – is one of the key benefits of physical activity, and of course as your child progresses, her enjoyment increases.

- **Sociability**: Having good interaction with peers and coaches and sharing her experiences with others is all part of the fun.

- **Being out there**: The final ingredient in the happiness equation is actually being in the outdoor environment.

The only downside to this is that the feel-good effects don't last forever, so you have to do the activity regularly to reap the rewards of increased happiness.

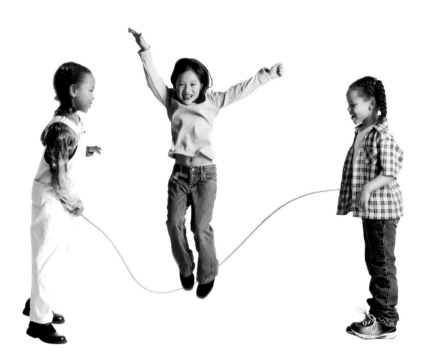

fact *An Australian study showed that doing regular, pleasurable physical activity in a social environment actually made unhappy people less neurotic and more extrovert.*

EVERY LITTLE HELPS

If your child (and perhaps the whole family) currently leads a sedentary lifestyle then organised exercise programmes are not necessarily the best place to start when you commit to being more active. In fact, anything that gets your child moving is an activity, so your first step is simply to encourage your child to replace some of his or her inactivity with activity (see Chapter Three for ideas). With positive reinforcement, sensitive handling and support from you, your child will soon start to feel that she is succeeding – and will want to enjoy that 'feel good' factor more and more.

Motivating your child

Knowing the facts is not the same as finding what will motivate your particular child to get active. After all, every parent knows that children fly in the face of common sense. Although you can point out that being active is fun, will improve her skills and help her to gain self-confidence and pleasure (because the experts have proved it), this is not convincing enough for the average child – and certainly won't wash with a teenager.

Bear in mind that, although it may be easier with a child who is naturally interested in sport or a good athlete, any child can be motivated. Obviously, every child is an individual and will respond to a different approach or mix of styles. Some need a great deal of praise, others react well to goal setting – you will best know your child's temperament and will be able to cherry pick from the following motivational suggestions to find what is right for your child:

Make sure it's fun

Finding that special 'fun' activity that appeals specifically to your child can be the catalyst for a lifetime of physical fitness. Often it is an activity that your child finds she is good at – but the overriding principle is that she enjoys it.

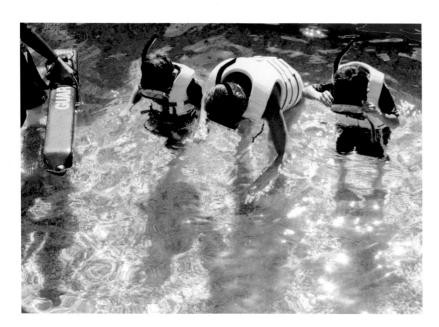

If it's an activity that you participate in as a family, then obviously, you must also enjoy it. As we have seen, parents who enjoy physical activity are good role models and their children are more likely to participate in physical activities themselves. (You will find more information on finding the right activity for your child and choosing clubs etc. in Chapter Four.)

Keep it varied

Throughout the week your child needs to perform a variety of different physical activities that do not just involve sport. Simply being active in various ways is the key. For example, walking to a friend's house, kicking a ball about with mates on the green, walking the dog, free play in the garden, dancing to music videos, doing chores, attending clubs and sports classes – all these pastimes will help your child to have a more active and healthy lifestyle.

Variety is also the key in terms of finding the right sport for your child. She cannot know what she excels at or what she particularly enjoys if she hasn't tried a multitude of different activities.

Rather than worry that your child cannot stick at anything, allow her to give a sport a try for a reasonable period and, if it's not for her, let her replace it with another activity. View it as a step along the way to finding a lifelong pleasure. As children grow, the activities that they enjoy and feel competent doing will change. One thing is for sure – if she feels sport is a burden she will give it up at the first opportunity.

Horses for courses

You should be sensitive to your child's tastes – perhaps she will prefer individual sports such as swimming or gymnastics rather than team activities. Seek out non-competitive activities for children who dislike the pressure of competition. Start with what you already know she likes. If she hated the school swimming gala but loves the pool on holiday, let her go to free swim sessions at the local pool but avoid lessons or swimming clubs. (See Chapter Four for more advice on finding the right activity for your child.)

> **tip** **A cautionary word**: while your child is finding her chosen sport, don't rush in and buy expensive kit, specialist clothing and equipment. Garages and lofts across the land are heaped to the rafters with discarded tennis rackets, martial arts outfits and junior golf clubs – so, until your child commits to a sport that you know she enjoys, borrow the clothing and equipment wherever possible, or make do with something suitable in the wardrobe (as long as this isn't a bar to her fitting in).

Be realistic

Your child probably will not seek out activities on her own. It is up to you to help her discover new and exciting activities that will fit in with her schedule and lifestyle.

Although we all hope that our children will shine in their endeavours, realistically, very few children become power athletes. As long as she is enjoying taking part in sport and activity she will be fit, healthy and happy – which is what we should all wish for our children.

fact *When you and your child are under pressure your brains release various stress-inducing chemicals. Exercise reduces the impact of these chemicals. Moreover, it provokes your body to release dopamine, endogenous opiates and serotonin – the chemicals that give us our sense of well-being. So if your child is feeling stressed or cheesed off – go out for a bike ride or take a bat and ball in the back garden and watch her buck up.*

ENCOURAGING PARTICIPATION IN SPORT

- **Reinforce the message that she doesn't have to be 'the best'**: Being part of a team, wearing team colours, sharing in the associated social activities and enjoying playing the game is what counts.

- **Offer encouragement**: When she performs well, make sure you tell her so. Praise hard work, getting up after a knock etc – look for the good in each game and give her positive feedback on it.

- **Praise effort, not outcome**: Remember to praise the effort she put in and the progress she has made rather than focussing on the scoreline or whether she won or lost.

- **Limit sedentary activity**: If she has unlimited access to sofa, TV remote, games console or computer there is little incentive to get up and go. Help her to make time for sport by limiting sedentary activities.

Combating negativity

If your child has always believed that she is no good at sport, that she can't run or that outdoor activity is for other kids but not her, then you must help her to overcome this lack of self belief.

It is a good practice to get your child into the habit of examining how she reacts to negative situations and feelings. Many kids are unaware that they can turn a situation such as missing one catch in cricket or rounders into 'I'm pathetic at sport', and from there it is a short step to 'I can't succeed at anything.' It is a good skill, not only for physical activity but also for life in general, to be able to turn negative 'self messages' such as these into positive 'self talk'.

How your child talks to herself in her head conditions her to believe things about herself. If she has convinced herself that she's 'not sporty' then she will behave accordingly, avoiding activity and shunning sporty friends. With your encouragement, and a bit of practice in positive 'self talk', she can start to anticipate potentially difficult situations. If we continue the scenario of the missed catch above, you could encourage her to think about a desirable outcome and to prepare a positive strategy before the inter-form rounders event that's coming up. Perhaps she can say to the PE teacher, 'I'm working on my catching but, until it's up to scratch, perhaps I could be bowler or back-stop for the tournament.'

Thinking positively can help build self-esteem and help your child to develop a strong self-image. Believing in her own ability to make a meaningful contribution in some way will help her in her pursuit of a healthier lifestyle.

tip

'Whether you think you can, or you think you can't, you'll be right.'

Henry Ford

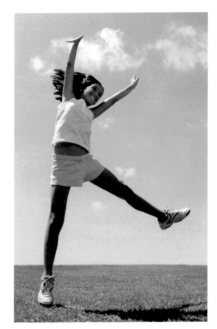

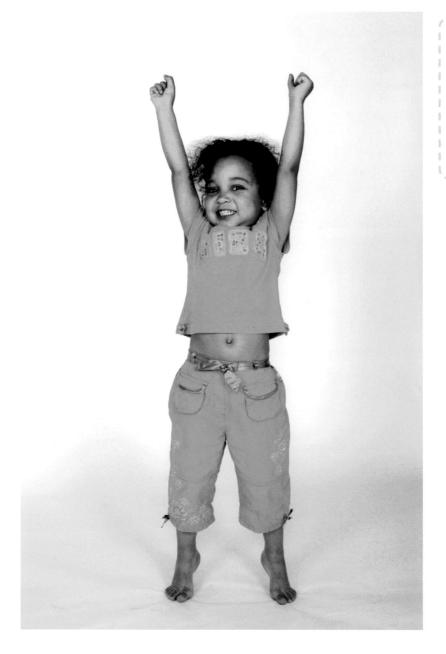

tip *Generally speaking, younger children are motivated by things that will make them like their super-heroes – taller, stronger, smarter, while older kids are more motivated by things that will improve appearance or sports performance.*

> **tip** One of the tools in your child's self-esteem armoury could be the use of affirmations. Used in many Eastern philosophies, these are positive statements that you tell yourself about your ability or your wishes. They should be said out loud and with conviction. For example, while taking her morning shower, your daughter might chant:
>
> **'I can do anything if I want it enough.'**
> **'I am sticking to my new activity plan.'**
> **'I like being active.'**
> **'I am fitter and healthier.'**
> **'I look and feel great.'**
>
> I'll leave the rest to her imagination and her own agenda but, suffice to say, telling yourself positive things is a great way to boost self-esteem.

Answering her fears

For many children, particularly those who are non-sporty or overweight, the thought of starting to participate in more sport or activity is fraught with anxieties, perhaps based on past experiences or, more often, on imagined fears. Common concerns include:

- I won't be able to do it.
- It's going to hurt.
- I'll never get to watch my favourite TV programmes any more.
- I'll have to work really hard.
- It will be boring.
- I'll look stupid.
- I'll be rubbish.
- The other kids will laugh at me.

Rather than dismiss these concerns as nonsense (because they may be very real to your child), be reassuring. Explain that things will be different for the whole family but that any changes in routine will be manageable and flexible. Discuss her fears, reassure her and encourage her to take a positive approach.

Although you are being sympathetic, you must also be firm. She has to realise that you are firm in your resolve that the family as a whole are bringing about changes towards a fitter and healthier lifestyle, and that being more active is not optional. Then you must lead by example.

Empathise by being active together

Peter Mackreth, Senior Lecturer in Physical Activity and Obesity Management at Leeds Metropolitan University and co-founder of their Residential Weight Loss Programme (commonly known in the press as 'The Fat Camp'), also runs community based programmes. He says,

'In the Community Projects, we get parents to set goals for themselves and their lifestyle. It's time for mum and dad that is social but also physical – perhaps something like salsa dancing. It shows the kids that physical activity is important to the parents and it makes the kids want to do it also.'

In Mackreth's experience, the majority of families with weight issues won't do any family activity together at all. He cannot stress strongly enough the significant role parents can play in this. He says, 'Role modelling is so important. If you value yourself, it will benefit your child too. It's good for kids to see their mum and dad doing something for themselves that's also healthy and sociable.'

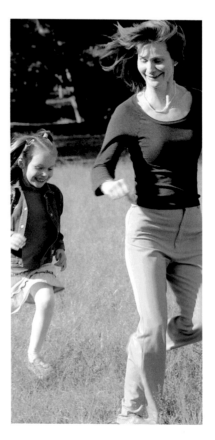

Although your child will undoubtedly protest at your exhortation to do something together – we've always walked as a family every weekend and our boys still groan when we say we're going out, even though they love it once they are outside – as she begins to realise that you are serious and determined, each time you say 'come on, we're going on a family bike ride' or whatever it happens to be, her protests will not be as long-winded, loud or adamant. And, once she's out with you, she will almost certainly enjoy the family activity, especially if you make sure it's something fun. Eventually, you may just get away with a withering look (if you're lucky) when you say, 'let's go!'

SELF-IMAGE

Non-sporty, lethargic or overweight kids are less likely to find acceptance from their peers and are more likely to develop a negative self-image, which can undermine feelings of self-worth and self-confidence.

If your child has become accustomed to believing that she is uncoordinated, rubbish at sport or generally too fat to participate, then you can start by dispelling these myths and promising positive results.

Building more activity into your child's life can counteract the negative emotions associated with poor self-image. Firstly, regular activity will increase the amount of endorphins – the body's natural mood enhancers – released in the body, which will help your child to feel happier.

Secondly, the resulting changes in your child's body from more exercise will help her to feel good about herself and to improve her self-image.

The couch potato

Don't despair if your child is non-sporty, unenthusiastic or perhaps overweight – there are still ways to motivate them and get them off the couch.

Be specific

Beware of falling into the parents' 'sanctimonious' trap. If you don't know what that is, see if the following example sounds familiar. You innocently say to your kids who are playing on the computer, 'It's such a lovely day. I can't believe you kids want to stay in this stuffy room. Why don't you go outside and get some exercise?' In fact, what your child hears is 'Nag, nag, nag', and what she thinks is, 'Why are you always preaching at me and telling me what to do?' Basically kids want to self-determine on these matters and to have a degree of choice. So that's what you give them – or so it seems.

Rather than whining on about nebulous notions of doing something, give them some much-desired control over which activity they do. Rather than saying, 'It's nice, shouldn't you be outside?' you say, 'The computer is going off in 5 minutes. Do you want to go swimming, cycling or meet some friends in the park to play frisbee?'

Peer pressure

In the above scenario, don't be surprised if your child chooses the latter option because most kids are keen to be involved in the activities that their friends are doing. Peers are hugely important, especially once kids hit the secondary school years, so it's always a good motivator to offer activity that involves meeting up with another child. You can even get your youngster motivated by allowing her to organise a group of friends to do some fun and challenging activity together such as paintballing, a game of rounders or a football

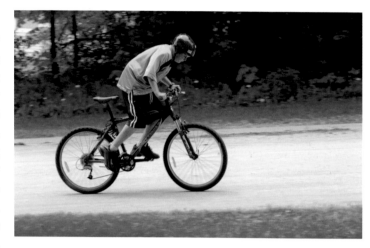

match in the park – parents of course have to be supportive in terms of getting children to and from such events if they are not old enough for independent travel (and, where applicable, cough up the necessary cash).

Required viewing?

One of the biggest enemies of getting children off the couch is the ubiquitous availability of in-home entertainment. Most families now have televisions in several rooms if not every room of the house, and kids have their own computers, games consoles and sound systems. Television shows such as soap operas and reality TV are the subject of endless discussions at school and, naturally, your child doesn't want to be left out. They are essential viewing. Similarly, having experience of the latest computer games is also vital if your child wants to be able to converse creditably with her peers. And, basically, all kids want to fit in.

To this end, youngsters can spend an inordinate number of hours shut away in a separate room in front of a screen. Often the curtains are drawn to create a numbing womb-like environment where they are unaware of the passage of time. Is it any wonder that they are reluctant to leave their cosy sanctuary to rush outside for some physical activity?

The first step to motivating the couch potato is to ration the TV and computer. Not only will this cut down on the amount of time spent in sedentary activity, but it will limit her exposure to the negative effects of TV commercials that target kids with the latest high-energy, low-nutrient snacks, cereals and fizzy drinks.

fact Scary small-screen statistics

- *Experts recommend that children under two should not be allowed to watch any TV or videos/DVDs. Over two-years-old, a child should watch no more than 1 or 2 hours a day and that allowance also includes time spent on computer/video games.*
- *The food industry spends £800 on advertising for every £1 spent by the Government on healthy eating education. Which message do you think is getting through?*
- *While watching television, the body's metabolic rate (the speed it burns calories) is even slower than its normal resting (or base) metabolic rate. So, bizarrely, watching TV is more fattening than quietly reading a book!*
- *According to The UK 2000 Time Use Survey up to the age of about 14, boys and girls watch a similar amount of television, although it rises from around 2 hours per day to nearer 3 hours at the age of 15.*

Understanding your child's mentality

Films such as *Freaky Friday* in which a battling mother (Jamie Lee Curtis) and teenage daughter (Lindsay Lohan) wake up inside each other's body one morning – to hilarious effect – are highly entertaining but, if it were possible, this would be a useful trick for the average parent because it would give us some insight into our children's lives.

Yet, even without the benefit of body exchange, it's a pretty sure bet to say that your youngster does not think the same way you do. She doesn't worry about her long-term health and does not share your concerns. When you were 15, did you worry about how you would be feeling when you were 50? Probably not. Don't forget that to a 15-year-old 21 is old, and anything beyond is simply unimaginable. So, nagging your child or adolescent to get active in order to avoid a heart attack in her sixties is not going to have any persuasive effect at all.

Fight fire with fire

To motivate a Key Stage 2 or secondary-school-aged child, you must meet her more than half way and try to understand her environment and the way she thinks. Paradoxically, the television could be one of the best ways to do this.

LOOKING THE PART

Another obstacle to becoming more active, especially for some girls, is whether or not they have the right clothing and exercise gear. It sounds ridiculous to most parents, but to image-conscious kids, the right look is essential.

I'm not advocating that you rush out and buy £100 trainers just to make your child feel more inclined to be seen outside, but allowing her to choose the sports clothes that make her feel appropriate and comfortable can make all the difference to her enthusiasm for being active.

When she is watching her rationed television programmes, a fair number of which will probably centre around reality shows and soaps, you can comment on the participants – noting that the fit, confident ones come across well. Get her feedback, too.

Similarly, you can do the same with your child's magazines. Obviously, you don't have to read them from cover to cover but if there's a celebrity on the front that your daughter thinks is cool, then you can drop into the conversation that you happen to know that the celeb in question keeps trim by using yoga and going to the gym. Appealing to your youngster's vanity and love of the rich and famous can be a powerful motivator.

However, appealing to her sense of style is something of a double-edged sword. Although you know that looking good is important to her, you certainly don't want to contribute any more than you have to towards the cult of celebrity or to encourage your child to aspire to the unrealistic ideal of an artificially thin, airbrushed model or celebrity. Nor do you want her to become self-obsessed and narcissistic. Rather, what you're trying to do is to talk to her in terms she'll understand and to use the things that she cares about and values as examples of why she should get off the couch.

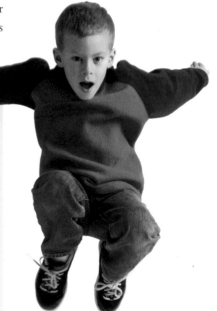

ICONIC APPEAL

In January 2007, Muhammad Ali launched a range of low-calorie children's snacks in the USA to coincide with his 65th birthday. The products are designed to encourage teenagers to 'eat like champions, walk like kings', and Ali is hoping that he can use his iconic status to help to teach children better eating habits.

The three-times World Heavyweight boxing champion says on his GOAT (Greatest Of All Time) website:

'It's time to pass on the values, beliefs and principles that made me a champ to the next generation of champions. I believe that better nutrition and respect for mind and body will give everybody today the opportunity to be the best they can be.'

One of Ali's prime motivators is his concern about the USA's increasingly overweight youth, of which he has first-hand experience – his 15-year-old son, Sadi, weighs more than him.

Curbing screen time

Here are some more ways to discourage your child from spending vast amounts of time in front of a screen, in isolation, and on her bottom:

- **Limit the number of television sets**: If you have a TV in every room, you are tacitly encouraging your child to slope off and watch TV on her own, which cuts down the amount of communication between a family and is the enemy of activity.

- **Make family mealtimes sacrosanct**: I know it's hard when members of the family have different commitments and schedules to follow, but eating together at the table gives the whole family an opportunity to communicate and gives you a chance to control what food your child is consuming. Eating supper on a tray in separate rooms watching different TV programmes or DVDs is a bad habit to slip into. It promotes snacking and grazing because eating while watching becomes habitual.

- **Lead by example**: If you and your partner also grab meals on the run or in front of the TV, your kids will not see it as anything exceptional. Even if you meet some resistance on the family meals idea, you and your partner should endeavour to sit down and eat together – that is the greatest inducement for your kids to join you.

- **No go areas for snacking**: If you make a rule that snacks and drinks cannot be consumed in bedrooms, or outside the kitchen – or whatever works for your household – you are making it harder for your child to simply stay put on the sofa surrounded by comfort food and drinks and with no incentive to move.

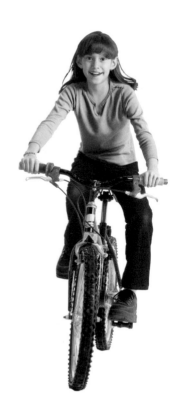

> ## tip TEEN EXERCISE
>
> *If your teenager is struggling to fit exercise into her busy schedule, you can help. Try to:*
>
> - *plan active outings as a family.*
> - *offer active family holidays.*
> - *continue to be a role model by being active and exercising yourself.*
> - *discourage watching too much TV or playing computer games in her rare spare time.*
> - *recommend lifetime sports such as swimming, running, tennis or cycling, rather than team activities, which she can practise and enjoy anywhere and on her own.*
> - *buy home exercise equipment or pay for a gym membership.*
> - *ease the problems by offering to drive to physical activity commitments.*
> - *encourage a part-time job that will reduce the amount of time that she spends in sedentary pursuits at home.*

Loss of interest in sport and physical activity

Throughout their lives, boys tend to spend more time on sporting activities than girls. The largest differences are for 12 to 13 year olds, where boys spend over 30 minutes per day longer than girls on sporting activities – with roughly 55 minutes a day spent participating in sport. Girls' interest in sport often wanes drastically when they go to secondary school, whereas boys' sporting activities don't tend to plummet until they hit 15 to 16 years old.

So, is there anything you can do if your once sporty youngster decides to give it all up? Unfortunately, the loss of interest in sport often coincides with a greater interest in teenage social activity. What's worrying for the parents of kids who turn their backs on sport is that research shows that those kids who continue in sport are less likely to take up smoking and drinking to excess.

> # fact *A US survey found that by the age of 11, more than half of children have left organised sport. The main reasons cited were:*
> - *It ceased to be fun.*
> - *It became too competitive.*
> - *I didn't have enough time to play.*

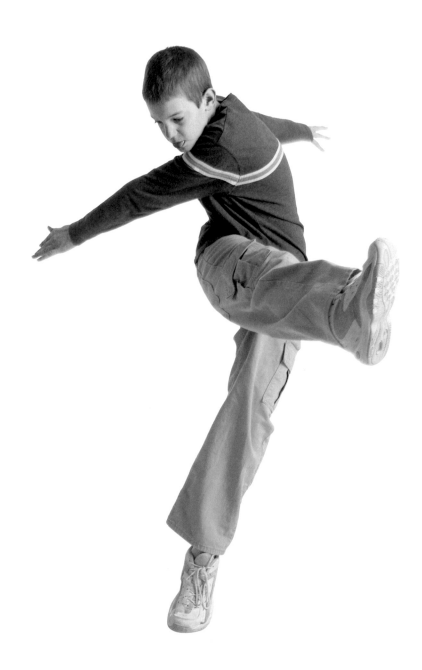

> **tip** *Quitting sport is more often than not a sign of your child's age and new interests, but occasionally it can be a sign of depression. If your child strikes you as being sad much of the time and she has lost interest not only in sport but also in other activities that she used to enjoy, it may be worth talking to your child's doctor. (For more information on signs of depression, see Chapter Six.)*

Nagging and dire health warnings will not work. In fact, a new approach is called for if you want to get your child back on track. Here are a few suggestions that might do the trick:

- **Address reasons for giving up**: It may be that your child is caving in to peer pressure and giving up on sport because she wants to fit in, even though she still enjoys it. However, if there is a valid reason, for example she loves gymnastics but hates the competitions, then supply the solution that keeps her at it, i.e. move her to a non-competitive class.

- **Try something new**: It may simply be that her existing sport or activity no longer excites her. In which case, let her try something new and thrilling. What about something completely different – archery, skateboarding, cheerleading – whatever appeals. Encourage her to give it a fair crack of the whip, though, because very often the first few attempts at a new activity are fairly disastrous.

- **Gym**: The gym is no longer the sole preserve of 'ladies who lunch' and bodybuilders. Most gyms and health clubs now offer classes and guided gym sessions specifically tailored to 12-year-olds and above. This can be a good option for the non-athlete who hates sports and the great outdoors but is body-conscious. (See box on page 33 for what to look for).

- **Home equipment**: For those who lack the motivation to participate in activities outside the house, or are extremely shy, some simple, inexpensive home equipment could be the answer. Our boys' rarely pass up the chance to do a couple of chin-ups when they pass the bar fitted to George's bedroom doorway – and neither can their friends when they visit. Alternatively, think about free weights, ab-flexors, exercise bands, Swiss balls or, if money is not an issue, then an exercise bike, rowing machine or treadmill could be ideal. All of these pieces of equipment can be used in front of the TV or while listening to music for the die-hard couch potatoes.

- **Gadgets and gizmos**: We live in a high-tech age and our children are born understanding how to operate technology. If you have a techno-wiz in the family, exercise gadgets and gizmos might be just the thing to add an incentive to activity. How about a pedometer? This device is worn at your child's waist and it counts each step she takes. It can also be calibrated (usually by the child rather than the technophobe parent) to measure the distance your child travels. Similarly, a mini bicycle computer can keep kids pedalling for hours at a time.

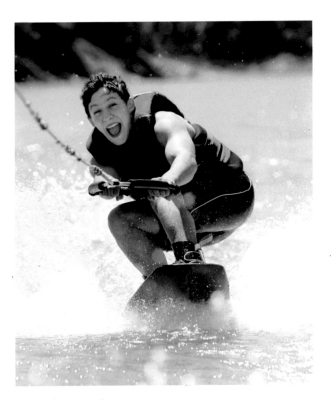

- **Book a court**: Why not book a badminton court and ask your daughter, her friend and her mother (preferably someone you know) to join you for a game. It's sociable and fun and could become a regular fixture. Tired of being a touchline mum, always watching her children's activities – particularly Libby's netball fixtures – our neighbour Catherine decided to take the initiative and get active. She books a netball court once a week and sends out a general invitation to Libby's friends, her own friends and other mums – and then there's a mixed generation netball match each week, which is great fun. Anyone can turn up whenever they like and it's become something of a social must in our neck of the woods, with the added bonus that it gets you fit.

- **Keep an activity log**: Sometimes the shock of seeing how little she does in the way of activity can be enough to startle your child into action – particularly if the whole family takes part and she's lagging way behind other members of the family.

- **Social appeal**: Ask your child to join you in some healthy pursuit and they may balk at the offer. Ask her if she wants to tag along while you meet some friends for a tango evening – or should you book a babysitter? – and she's more likely to jump at the chance. A bit like hiding vegetables in a casserole, disguising activity in a social environment is a handy guise.

■ **Buy a dog**: This is not a solution that should be undertaken lightly. However, many children and teenagers love dogs and having a puppy of their own can be a good way of getting every member of the family out walking. Obviously, there are other considerations and, if you go down this route, your child must be prepared to commit to her share of the walking, just as you must be prepared to enforce this commitment (with a little latitude obviously). A dog is definitely more work, but ownership can be hugely rewarding and a real fitness incentive.

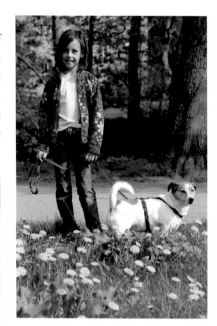

GYM'LL FIX IT

When looking for a gym that your child can attend, there are a few things to consider:

■ Make sure the health club or gym you are considering offers a family membership discount or special rates for students and under-21s, which can make this a much more affordable option. Off-peak membership is also worth asking about since your child will probably visit after school most often, which fits into that membership bracket.

■ Seek out classes that are specifically tailored to kids and those that are for parents and children (there are usually a limited number of places for children in these classes because of the statutory requirements for the ratio of staff to children so it is advisable to book early to avoid disappointment, as they say.)

■ Don't limit yourself to gym and studio-based classes. There should be a good selection of other activities on offer such as Thai kickboxing, salsa, aquaerobics, circuit training etc. One of these is bound to appeal to you and your child.

■ Look at high school and college gyms – some are opening up to outside customers as a way of raising revenue. It's often a cheaper option than the commercial equivalents.

■ Pick a local gym or one that is accessible by public transport from your home/child's school. If it's a lot of hassle to reach, or she has to depend on a lift from you, she won't make the most of her membership.

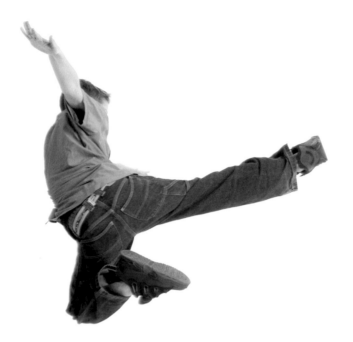

Q&A

Question: My 11-year-old son is uncoordinated and nervous. He has not yet found a physical activity that suits him, but he is not totally resistant to being active. In fact, he'd like to be a member of a team but doesn't feel that he's good enough to be selected. What might suit him?

Answer: Your son can choose from numerous activities that do not involve competitive team sport. Perhaps he should look for a group activity rather than an individual sport so that he is participating with others but not competing against them. For example, martial arts, swimming clubs and circuit training or resistance training.

   If he would still like to enjoy the sociable aspect of team sport, he could simply attend training and make it clear that he doesn't want to play in matches. Alternatively, he could enjoy 'team spirit' by volunteering to be part of the management and administration team.

Q&A

Question: My 12-year-old daughter plays for a team but her enjoyment of the sport is being ruined because the coaches do not encourage her effort since she is not one of the 'stars'. I don't want her to be put off just because she's not a superstar. What can I do?

Answer: It is worth having a private word with the coaches. You may wish to point out to them how your daughter feels or you may prefer to ask them how your child can improve her skills and what they can do to help her impove.

It is very difficult to be critical of coaches when so many are giving up their free time without payment. However, the overall sporting experience for your daughter should be positive. If she is still enjoying the opportunity this team provides for exercise, fun and teamwork, that's the main objective. If this is not the case, and things do not improve after your talk with the coaches, then I would consider finding another team who value effort and participation more highly.

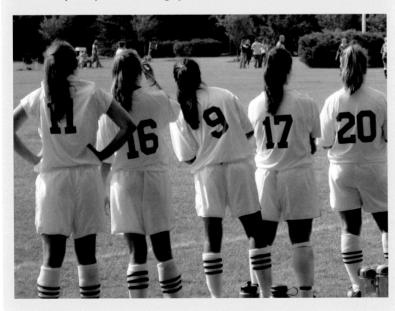

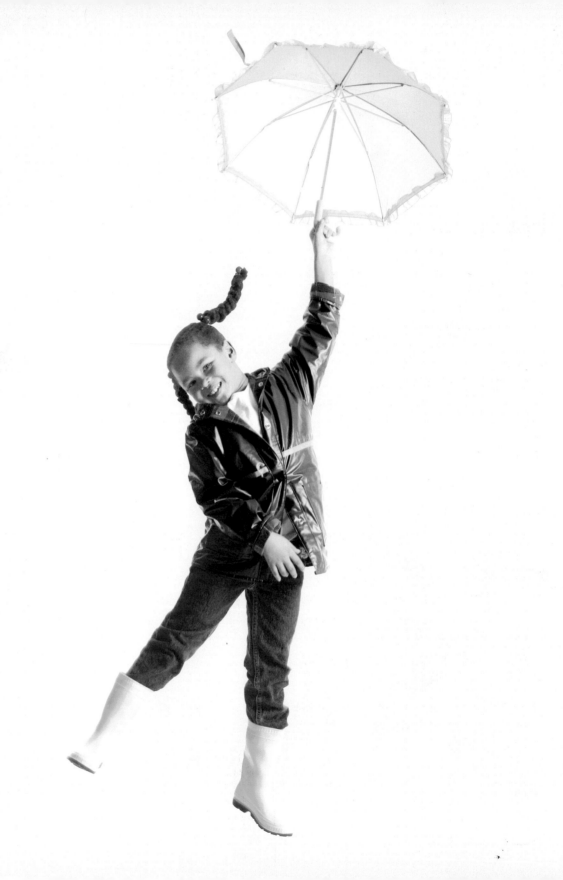

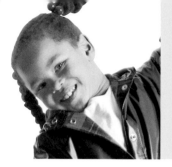

3 getting active

Fitting fitness in

Of course, I recognise that it is not easy for time-strapped, busy modern parents to fit anything else into an already over-stuffed family schedule, but it is not impossible.

You don't have to be out there indulging in strenuous exercise five days a week – just getting out there and doing something that is fun with the kids sets an example and is an inspiration that children can adopt and carry into adulthood.

In the beginning, however, if you are not able to set aside time to do specific activities together as a family, then a good starting point is to simply grab every chance during your day to take the physically more demanding option. It sounds basic but it is an effective way to build more activity into a hectic lifestyle. For example, you can:

■ take the stairs instead of the escalator or lift.

■ walk or cycle with your child to school.

■ If time doesn't permit the above option, then park the car a little further from school than normal and walk the last bit.

■ Instead of choosing the parking space nearest the supermarket, park further away and walk briskly to the shop.

■ Go about the daily household chores with gusto – vacuum at speed, put some elbow grease into the polishing and play your favourite dance CD while doing the dishes so you can bop while you mop.

■ If it is not your weekly shop, take a basket rather than a trolley.

■ Wherever possible, walk rather than drive. Often you could walk to a friend's house just as easily. Driving is often a habit.

These may seem like small and pointless measures but, by making a point of choosing the physical, healthier option over the sedentary choice, you are conditioning yourself and your family into a way of thinking that encourages activity and exercise and promotes greater activity.

fact *The proportion of school children spending less than 1 hour per week on physical education (PE) rose from 5 per cent in 1994 to 18 per cent in 1999.*

GETTING EVERYONE INVOLVED

With a little gentle persuasion – or you may have to resort to bribery – you can get the whole family involved in doing the household chores. In this way, exercise just happens without it being a big deal.

Remember, doing the ironing while watching the TV is more beneficial than sitting and watching the box. Vacuuming burns still more calories.

Here are some suggestions, but I am sure you and the family can come up with more of your own:

- Cleaning the car
- Vacuuming
- Mowing the lawn and weeding the garden
- Creating a vegetable patch
- Raking leaves
- Cleaning your room
- Pet husbandry, for example cleaning out rabbit hutches
- Shopping
- Walking the dog
- Clearing snow off the drive/path

Where do you start?

Your overall aim is to make activity an integral part of your family's life. Sometimes, though, the thought of getting each member of the family involved in daily exercise or regular sport is too overwhelming and getting started can seem like an insurmountable objective.

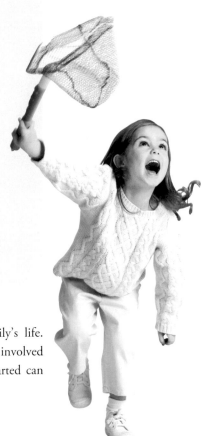

So, making small changes in your daily routines that will not alarm your child or cause major inconvenience to you is the best place to start. Introducing a family outing at weekends, or walking to visit friends rather than taking the car – small, unobtrusive steps that you increase incrementally. Eventually, you will be able to build up to a family routine that ensures everyone's good health and which may, or may not, eventually include sport and workouts!

As your family experiences the positive results of this change in routine, so it will help inspire you all to continue to be more active and to permanently adopt a healthier lifestyle. And once your kids get used to doing more as a family, so they will be more inclined to be active on their own initiative and under their own steam. Believe it or not, research shows that the vast majority of kids would be naturally physically active, given the opportunity, and you can build on this natural inclination.

One of the first steps is to make sure your home is conducive to your family and, in particular, your child being active. Have you thought about whether or not your home environment is an activity-friendly area?

Outdoor fun

Take a look in your garden. Is there a table and chairs for the fine weather? Some flower beds in need of attention? Maybe even a barbecue? Not much there to entice the kids though, is there?

Why not think about putting some age-appropriate items in the garden that will make being outside fun and tempting? For little kids, you could put in an inexpensive sandpit or paddling pool (this will obviously need supervising). Let them chalk a hopscotch pattern on the patio – it will keep them occupied for ages. A skipping rope is good for little ones and also invest in a longer rope for when friends come round – they can make up their own rhymes and games, or you can teach them the ones you learned in the playground all those moons ago. As for set pieces of equipment, a swing is always popular as are climbing frames and mini-football nets.

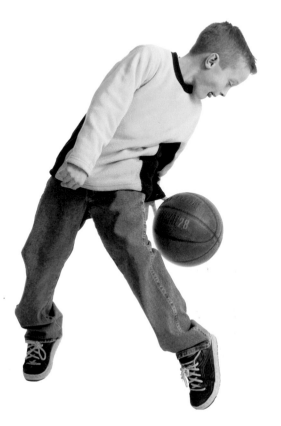

As he gets older, your child might enjoy climbing on a rope swing or ladder, but any equipment that is readily available to him and doesn't require hours of setting up will entice your child outside. A basketball hoop on the side of the house can keep older children occupied, as will a badminton net, croquet hoops or miniature golf set. Get some friends round for a volleyball match. If you don't have a net you can always improvise with a rope strung between two poles or trees. A string bag full of various sizes of ball from tennis to football, rugby to basketball will provide plenty of fun – and collecting them all up at the end of the day can be a fun activity, too!

It doesn't have to be an expensive item such as a climbing frame or trampoline. However, if budget and space permit, these big items are a good investment as a permanent piece of equipment that are enormously popular with older kids and that they do use (I can vouch for it). Perhaps such an item could replace the swing set as your child grows up and his needs and tastes change.

SUPERVISED PLAY

Most of the time, children can occupy themselves in free play quite happily if there are things in the garden to entice them. However, for those who are a little more reluctant to leave the house or who are not good self-starters, here are some ideas for games that require a leader – yes, that would be you (or you could rope an older brother or sister in – after all, it gets them out of the house and it could be a way for them to earn pocket money?)

- **Follow my leader**: Make it as energetic or gentle as you like. Just make sure you keep them on the move as you skip, hop, star-jump, dance and cartwheel around the garden.

- **Wacky races**: A great way to even the odds if you have a child who is not a natural athlete. Organise egg and spoon races, sack races, three-legged races, walking backwards races. The list is endless and provides hours of fun. Try to ensure each child wins a race, if possible. And for competitive kids, there are always good old running races.

- **Dodgeball**: This is a classic playground team game that is particularly popular with boys. The aim is to hit your opponents with the ball to eliminate them until there is one player left – and his team wins. Please note: although it's advisable to use a soft ball, it can still get out of hand without supervision.

- **Play-acting**: You tell the story and the children act it out. This is good for small children. You can make your imaginary tales as adventurous and wild as you like – kids love pretending to be animals, superheroes and monsters.

GET THEM OUT

If you don't have a garden then investigate where the nearest park is located, and make up a box or basket stuffed with exciting items, such as the following, to take with you whenever you go:

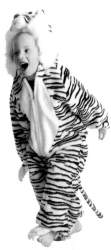
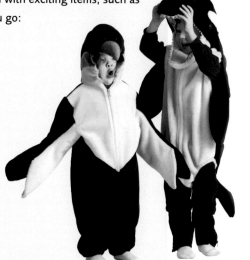

- Frisbee
- Bat and ball
- Football
- Baseball glove and mitt
- Kite
- Skipping ropes
- Hula-hoops
- Rollerblades
- Skateboard

Don't forget the bicycles. If it's too far to ride to the park, put the kids' bikes in the boot and then at least they can ride around the paths at the park when you get there. And there's always the enticement of the fabulous play equipment that so many parks now provide – swings, climbing frames, teeter-toys and monkey bars appeal to kids of all ages.

Indoor play

Making the inside of your home activity-friendly can be a challenge because most parents are understandably reluctant to have their ornaments and family heirlooms trashed by flying balls and boisterous play. That said, there are plenty of ways to encourage more physical alternatives to the ubiquitous television:

- Push back the furniture to make a dance area/space for imaginary play.
- A dressing up box – superheroes and princesses rarely sit still!

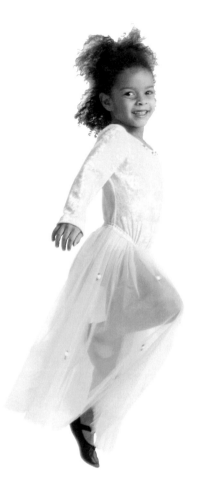

- A karaoke machine, or even a microphone and some musical instruments encourage performances that can become pretty energetic, particularly if your child's tastes veer towards rock 'n' roll rather than ballads.

- Balloons – using hands, bats, feet, the game is to make sure they don't touch the floor.

- A game of Twister™ gets kids and adults alike on the go – just be careful you don't crush your youngster when you topple.

- A hopscotch mat.

- A dartboard – there are child-safe versions for younger members of the family.

- Techno-kids will love the power-pad dance-mats, kickboxing or football games that translate your child's body movements on to the computer screen.

Indoors or outdoors, the aim is to provide as much opportunity and incentive as possible to get your child playing, moving and being active.

FITNESS FOR FUNKY FOLK

Dance is a great way to get active without even realising that you're exercising. It's just such fun – and something your child can do at home with nothing but a CD player and floor space, or she can do with friends or in a class. For those who like it funky, check out:

- Salsa – the heady mix of Latin American and Afro-Caribbean rhythms will get their bodies moving!.

- Belly dancing is great for toning up legs, bums, waist and hips – and it's great fun.

- If your child was hooked on BBC One's *Strictly Come Dancing*, sew on some sequins and get her down to the ballroom dancing studio.

- And if the stage beckons, why not suggest tap dancing for any budding Ginger Rogers.

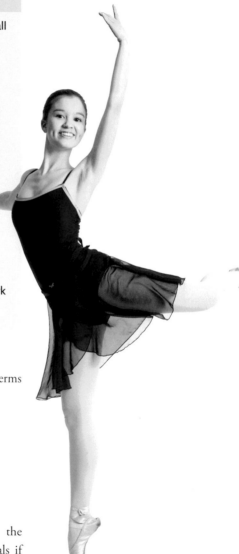

FIRST STEPS

At the beginning, it may be hard to rein in your natural enthusiasm to put all you've read into practice but remember:

- **Pace yourself**: Fired up with enthusiasm, it's tempting to try to do everything at once and put all your ideas into action straight away. Rather, you should take one step at a time and only introduce a couple of changes at any one time to your family.

- **Positive outcomes**: Make sure your first goals are those that you can accomplish comfortably. That way, your child's early successes and accomplishments will form a positive foundation for future changes. Remember, success breeds success.

- **If it ain't broke don't fix it**: In other words, don't work on problems that your family doesn't have just because you've read about it. For example, don't waste time researching non-competitive team sports when he's perfectly happy thrashing it out with other kids. Instead, work on cutting down on the hours he spends playing on computer games.

Setting SMART goals

The acronym SMART is commonly used in management circles in terms of goal setting and it stands for:

S pecific
M easurable
A ttainable
R ealistic
T ime frame

This system might be seen more commonly in the boardroom than the playground, but your family is much more likely to meet its activity goals if you apply the SMART instrument when setting your objectives.

For each new activity that you plan, you should prepare the SMART way. Let's take the example that your child wants to walk more on a regular basis. You would think along the following lines:

Specific: Helps you to focus his efforts and to define what you are going to do.

- What will he need? Does he need new trainers or walking shoes?
- Where will he walk? Can he walk to and from school?
- Who with? Is he able to walk the dog on his own yet? Does he need someone to accompany him?

Measurable: Where possible, choose a goal with measurable progress. So 'I want to walk to school three days a week' is a measurable target, whereas 'I want to walk more often' is not.

Attainable: If you set goals that are too far out of your reach you probably won't commit to doing them. For example, if your son says he wants to do a 16-kilometre (10-mile) hike every weekend there's a good chance he's being over-ambitious. Perhaps committing to walk the dog every evening and to have a family walk on Sundays is something that will stretch him (and you) but, with some commitment, it is possible.

Realistic: By this, you should not think 'easy' so much as 'do-able'. A realistic activity plan should push your family's commitment and ability, but it shouldn't break your resolve or enthusiasm. Remember that goals that are too difficult set the stage for failure, but goals that are too low send the message to your family that you are not very committed or capable.

Time frame: Set a time frame for your goal. 'I want to be able to walk a mile in less than ten minutes by the time I'm ten' is a clear and sensible time target to work towards (hopefully when he's nine, not six!).

Fun family activities

As we have seen, if you want to keep your kids on the move, you have to lead by example – let them see you having fun while being active, and especially enjoying yourself when it comes to active family time together.

After-school clubs/activities and sports clubs are great for motivated, sporty or active kids but if your child is one of those who is unenthusiastic about physical activity, despite the best intentions on your part, signing the form, writing the cheque and packing them off to such organised activities will be met with huge resistance and is probably ultimately doomed to failure – particularly if he has shown no interest in the pastime to date. Coercion 'for the good of your health' won't work.

So, we're back to doing things together. The key, yet again, is enjoyment. There are two places to start:

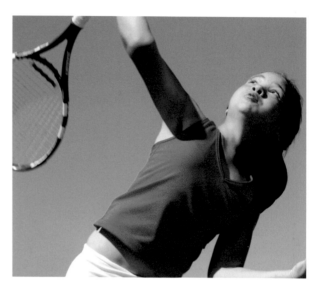

Doing something you enjoy

If you love playing tennis, then there is a very good chance that your child is going to want to give it a try, too. For the serious sporting parent, this can pose a problem because it means sacrificing some of your games to include your child in a way that is meaningful and not intimidating. Collecting balls for you while you play a match is not going to get him into the game. Similarly, giving him the benefit of your finest coaching skills will probably turn what could be a fun shared activity into a bore for him.

Make it fun – you could even invite a few of his friends along to share the court – and, if you desperately miss your competitive matches, book an extra session for adults at another time.

Doing something your child enjoys

Once you are aware of your child's interests and likes, you are well placed to find an activity that maximises this knowledge. For example, the boy who loves to play kick-ass computer games could well be enticed by a group ju-jitsu taster session at the local leisure centre (don't worry – most martial arts place heavy emphasis on the philosophy of self-control and restraint, not violence).

Similarly, a girl who is animal mad might like to take part in horse riding during a family holiday. And, if she enjoys it, learning to ride expends a surprising amount of energy. This is not, of course, a cheap hobby but for cash-strapped parents there are often schemes on offer whereby a child can muck out stables and groom their beloved horses for several weekends in order to earn a free ride on the 3rd or 4th weekend.

SIX OF THE BEST: GET WISE TIPS FOR INVOLVED PARENTS

Sadly, we've probably all seen examples of 'competitive parents' where kids are bullied into participating in a sport that holds no allure for them simply because the parent wants to relive his sporting experiences or because they want to bathe in their child's reflected glories.

This is one of the biggest turn-offs for a child and can lead to rebellion in teenage years, where the child rejects all sporting activity as a result. If you're reading this book, then it's very unlikely that you're the sort of unaware character who would resort to these bullying tactics but, even so, there are a few pitfalls to avoid when trying to induce your child to be more active:

1 Never force your child into an activity that holds no appeal for him, or compare him to active friends/cousins/boy next door.

2 Don't expect him to excel at an activity or sport simply because you were good at it at school. He is not a mini version of you.

3 Don't slob about at home after a hard day's work if you expect him to get out there and be active. Remember you're a role model.

4 Don't dwell on the fact that you have always hated PE and did everything in your power to get out of PE at school. Put that behind you because you have now got to make an effort to be positive about being active for the sake of your family's health.

5 Don't be too blatant. If you jump at every opportunity to get your child signed up for an activity, however unsuitable, he will soon pick up on your desperation to get him fit and will recoil. Worse still, in typical childlike fashion, he could also interpret your actions as, 'S/he doesn't like me how I am. I'm a disappointment.' Subtlety is the name of the game.

6 Don't resort to emotional blackmail when things aren't going to plan. If your child isn't sticking to any of the new activities, or still shows no sign of enthusiasm, frustration can lead to a 'do you know how much I've spent on this?' style knee-jerk reaction. Playing the 'after all I've done for you' card usually cuts no ice with youngsters and is, more often than not, counter productive – making him less likely to want to try something new next time.

Activity ideas

Now that you've started to:

■ take the physical option over the easy choice in your everyday lifestyle

■ incorporate some more activity into your own life

■ try to inspire your child to greater efforts in the forms of clubs or sporting participation. . .

here are some ideas for some alternative activities that your child might enjoy, either with or without the rest of the family:

- archery
- skateboarding
- fencing
- baton twirling and cheerleading
- ice skating
- ice hockey
- in-line skating
- mountain biking
- stunt biking
- horse riding
- golf.

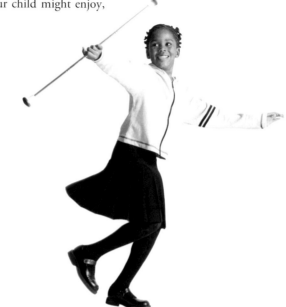

Happy holidays

As part of your drive to be more active as a family, why not swap your summer holiday lazing by the pool for an adventure holiday? It doesn't have to be high-adrenalin stuff. If bungee jumping and white-water rafting don't appeal look for something on the gentler side.

Sport holidays: Maybe a cycling trip through Provence, for example? Obviously choose somewhere that's not too hilly and where the company takes your luggage from location to location – and then you can take it as leisurely as you like.

Clubs: How about a Club holiday, such as Club La Santa or Club La Manga, where you are effectively having a poolside holiday with extra sports facilities and classes on offer?

Family specialists: There are family-holiday specialists, such as Mark Warner, who run summer and winter club holidays tailored to the needs of families. On such a break, a range of activities are available and there are clubs for the kids so they can go off and be occupied and entertained while you relax – but don't forget your resolve to be a role model!

BAD WEATHER ACTIVITIES

During the winter months, short, cold and/or rainy days and long, dark nights can see the best-intentioned families resorting to staying home. Rather than giving up on your good intentions you can prevent the kids from going stir-crazy with a little imagination.

Admittedly, a lot of these suggestions require some spare cash but it's a better health investment than another DVD rental or computer game, and you can also be inventive and come up with ideas that cost next to nothing if you put your thinking cap on:

- **Fitness and leisure centres**: Book a court for badminton or indoor tennis and play doubles. Why not sign up for a class in an activity that none of you has ever tried before and give it go – it might be something that you all enjoy. Most local leisure centres have a selection of classes ranging from table tennis and volleyball to martial arts and wall climbing.

- **Go swimming**: This doesn't have to be an activity solely reserved for warm weather.

- **Ice skating**: If the weather is bad, you might as well wrap up and get on the ice. Indoor rinks are open all year round and many cities now have outdoor rinks set up around the festive season, which are great family fun.

- **Museums**: Here is an activity that is not only good fun but also free and available in nearly every town in the country. Factual quizzes and trails can offer added interest value and keep your child on the move.

- **Aquariums and indoor nature centres**: Our local library has an aquarium in the basement that is free and my children still love it, despite having visited on numerous occasions.

- **Exercise classes and dance studios**: Everything from ballet to line dancing, yoga to hip hop is available – take your pick.

- **Indoor play areas**: Good fun for younger kids. They can kick off their shoes, launch themselves into the ball-pit and burn off some excess energy.

Skiing: In the winter, you could consider a skiing holiday where you are sure to have fun as a family – and you're active all day long in the most wonderful mountain setting. Again, there are family specialists such as Mark Warner, Ski Esprit and Ski Famille, but many of the big ski tour operators are also well geared up for family skiers.

Water sports: If you are a family of 'water babies', Plas Menai, the UK National Water Sports Centre in Wales, can give you a sample of just about

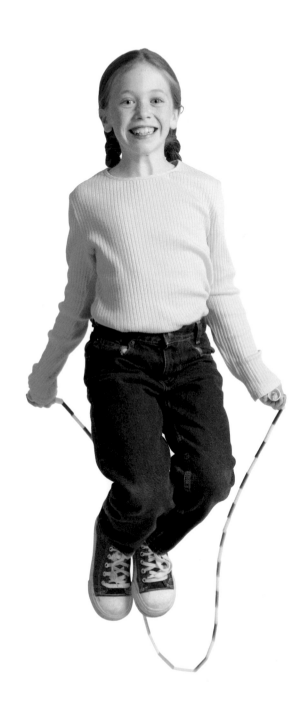

every water sport ever devised. They also run courses for children on their own or for families. And if this whets your appetite sufficiently (no pun intended), and you all love the water, a sailing cruise or canal boat holiday can be relaxing, but still keeps the family on the move and active in short bursts.

Adventure travel: Perhaps you want to ditch the poolside holiday for something more adventurous but don't want an activity holiday as such. Then why not look at Explore family holidays, or something similar, which offers a range of trips to exotic locations? Choose from holidays exploring the caves and castles of Slovenia, through island-hopping sailing tours of the Greek islands, to camel treks in the Moroccan deserts, and big-cat safaris in India and Africa.

Camping: If you're looking for more of a budget break, a camping holiday or beach holiday is the perfect solution for the active family. You can load the car up with bats and balls and games, and just being in the fresh air for a fortnight will get everyone in the mood for being active. If the weather let's you down, don't suffer under canvas – get out there and have a blustery walk along the cliff tops! Or go swimming in the rain – it feels great when you get out!

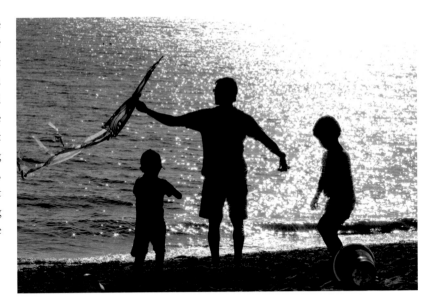

FITNESS BABYSITTERS

Increasing numbers of cash-rich, time-poor parents are hiring personal trainers to work out with their youngsters on a one-to-one basis.

Many of the parents who buy into this latest trend use personal trainers themselves, and see enlisting their services for their offspring (at a cost of around £30 an hour) as a logical investment in their family's fitness. Most argue that they don't have time to be active with their children themselves (although we know it can be done), so employing a 'fitness babysitter' is the next best thing.

One London-based personal training company now estimates that around one-quarter of their clients are children. However, not everyone agrees that personal training for children is such a good idea.

Some experts in the industry feel that this 'quick fix' solution for too little exercise is not the answer, and that exercising and adopting a healthier lifestyle as a whole family is a better option. Critics are also concerned about the lack of specialist training for personal trainers working with children (children must not do resistance training with weights because their tendons and ligaments haven't fully formed). They also contest that personal training is a poor substitute for free play or sport.

Those who support the new trend believe that one-to-one training can be a good way to boost sagging self-esteem and combat poor body image (which is a perennial problem with today's youth). Supporters also maintain that personal training educates children and gets them into the habit of exercising.

You will have to draw your own conclusions on this new development but, if you are tempted to use a personal trainer for your child, there are a couple of precautionary measures you should follow:

- Check that the personal trainer has insurance and is qualified.

- Has s/he been trained to work specifically with children? In August 2006, the YMCA – widely seen as the 'Gold Standard' for instructors – piloted a course called YMCA Fit Kids for fitness instructors who want to train children either on a one-to-one basis or in groups. Details can be found at www.ymcafit.org.uk or by phoning 020 7343 1850 and pressing 1 for Customer Services.

- Has s/he been police checked to work with children? (See Criminal Records Bureau www.crb.gov.uk or www.disclosure.gov.uk for information about the disclosure service).

Cool stuff to do for teenagers

By the time your child has reached his mid-teens, you are looking at a target of a minimum of three 20-minute sessions of exercise a week. Ideally, they should be getting closer to the adult target of 30 minutes physical activity each day but, realistically, teenagers have so many commitments on their time – from study to extra-curricular commitments and even part-time jobs – that it's small wonder they only want to text their friends and watch TV in their down time.

Many previously active kids have also dropped out of team sports (again, often because of time pressures), so activities to pique their curiosity and to get a wired teen on the move have to be exciting and unusual. As they would say in text-speak: So ParNts, herez some awsum ideas, init:

- Water sports such as windsurfing, canoeing, kayaking, rafting, sailing, bodyboarding, surfing, doughnuting and kneeboarding (where you get towed behind a powerboat, crossing the wake and carving around corners).

- Paintballing.

- Laser Tag (high-tech tag where you get to shoot your opponents with 'laser' guns).

- Tenpin bowling.

- Dance (salsa, hip-hop, flamenco plus more traditional – tap, jazz, line or ballroom).

- Snowboarding and skiing.

- Skateboarding and in-line skating.

- Archery.

- Fencing.

- Fitness classes such as kick-boxing, Pilates, yoga, Pace, aerobics.

- Gym classes such as circuit training, weight training etc.

- Rock climbing (indoor and outdoor).

- Outdoor sports such as mountain biking, hiking, orienteering and geocaching (see box on page 54).

- Beach games such as volleyball, hacky sacking and frisbee.

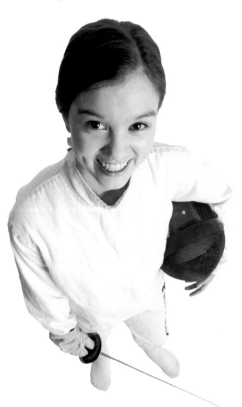

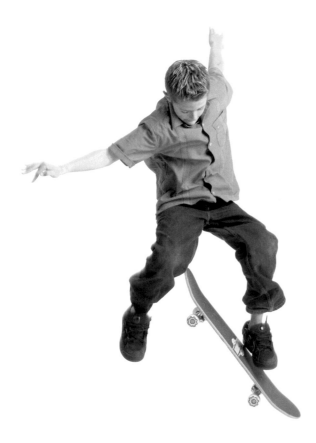

- Coasteering (wearing specialist climbing equipment, and under expert supervision, you pick your way along the bottom of a sea cliff – great fun and very wet!)

- Gorge walking and canyoning (you work your way up or down a river gorge, climbing waterfalls, crossing pools and negotiating objects.)

Many of the above activities are far from cheap. However, thrill-seeking teens are often happy to contribute towards the price if it means they get to sample some new and adrenalin-pumping activity. And, if they discover an activity that lights their fire, there are usually clubs available that make it more affordable long term.

GEOCACHING

Basically, geocaching is a high-tech version of hide-and-seek. Geocachers seek out hidden treasures utilising GPS coordinates posted on the Internet by those hiding the cache. Using a GPS unit (which can be bought for as little as £90 and used time and time again) you then trek out into the backwoods or urban jungles to find the hiding spot of the cache. Once discovered, geocachers follow a simple set of rules:

- Fill out the logbook.

- Take something out (people hide CDs, small toys, disposable cameras etc.)

- Put something back in.

- Return the cache, in the condition in which it was found, to the exact position it was found.

It can be as simple as walking to an open area at a local park or as difficult as searching for multiple locations to find the final prize. Some caches have even been planted on mountainsides or under water! It's growing and evolving as a new gaming activity every day.

Charles Newgas of Finger Technology explains its popularity: 'Parents have discovered that it's good fun and it gets you into the fresh air and away from the computer screen.' Geocaching is a gaming activity that appeals to a wide range of people. Young and old are getting involved. Families, gaming clubs, civic organisations and school groups are heading outdoors in search of hidden treasure.

Geocaching can be a great day out where you'll all get lots of exercise because sometimes getting to the caches involves quite a hike. Remarkably, because of the high-tech element, even previously lethargic teenagers are keen to be involved in a high-tech treasure hunt.

Geocaching started on 3 May 2000. By the end of June 2006 there were:

- 281,971 active caches hidden worldwide in total

- 222 countries with geocaches placed

- 11,679 active caches hidden in the UK alone

- 180,010 'finds' logged in the UK during one week in June 2006.

(Definition and data courtesy of
www.fingertech.co.uk)

tip **PREVENTING INJURY**

For those who have recently increased their activity levels after years of being sedentary, there are certain precautions to prevent injury that are worth considering:

- *Despite initial enthusiasm that you do not want to quash, don't let your child train or practice for too many hours at the beginning.*
- *Make sure your child learns the correct and safe technique from a qualified instructor, if possible.*
- *Use the correct equipment, if appropriate.*
- *Teach your child how to recognise the difference between muscle soreness, from repeating unfamiliar movements, and pain.*
- *Make sure your child knows when to stop. Kids of a competitive disposition can push themselves too far rather than lose face and stop before another participant.*

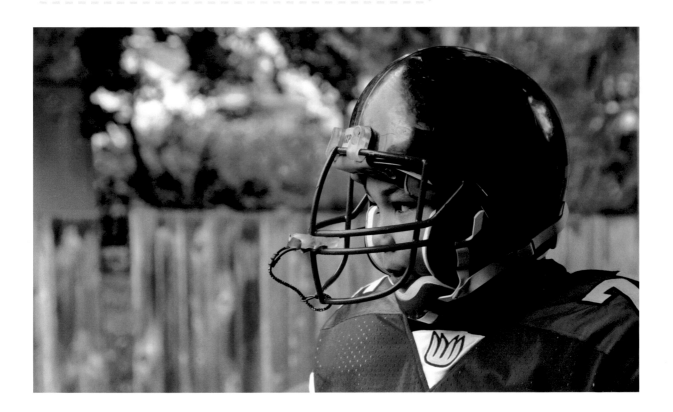

Q&A

Question: My 11-year-old son has never played in a team sport before and not really shown much interest in any competitive sports at all, despite the fact that many of his friends are sporty. Recently, he has said that he wants to join a junior football team that plays in a local league. Is he too old to start and how can I prepare him?

Answer: It's great that your son is keen to join a team and to play a sport regularly. At this level, where most teams train once a week and play a match once a week, he probably won't need any special training or fitness preparation. If the team is more serious than this then a word with the coach about whether additional fitness and skills training is advisable might be worthwhile.

It is worth checking out the standard and attitude of this team. If they have been playing in a league together for some time, they may be serious about getting good results. A relaxed atmosphere with friendly competition might be more suitable for your son as a novice to team sports – if the atmosphere is fiercely competitive, and the skill levels high, he might be demoralised if he has to earn a place on the team through merit or, worse, if his teammates make him feel that he is letting down the side due to his lack of experience.

Question: At what age should my child start competitive team or individual sports?

Answer: It is recommended that you don't start a child in competitive sports before the age of seven or eight. Before that age most children do not have the necessary skills, the attention span or the concentration required for organised sport.

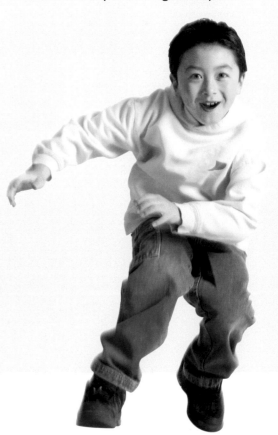

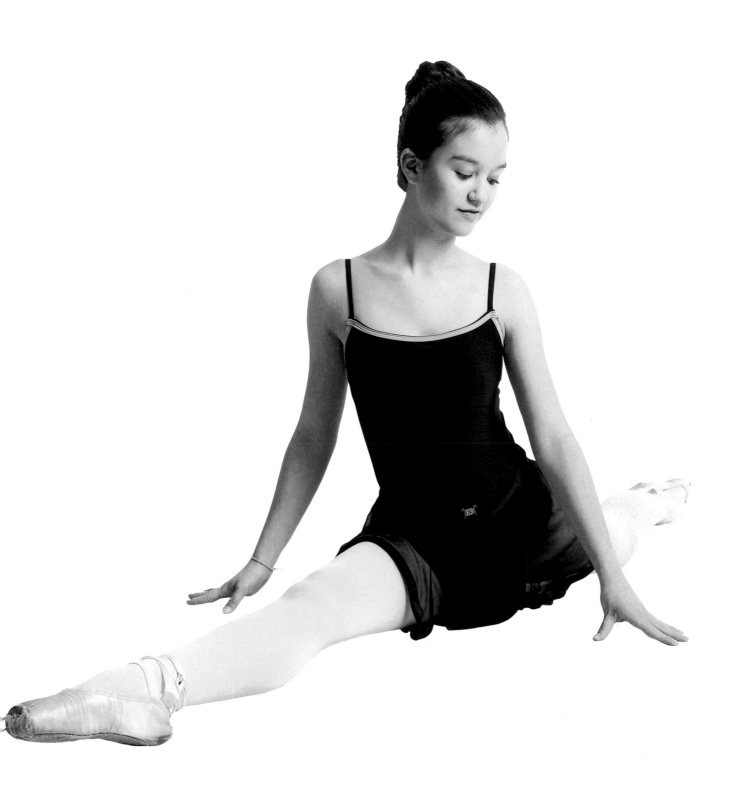

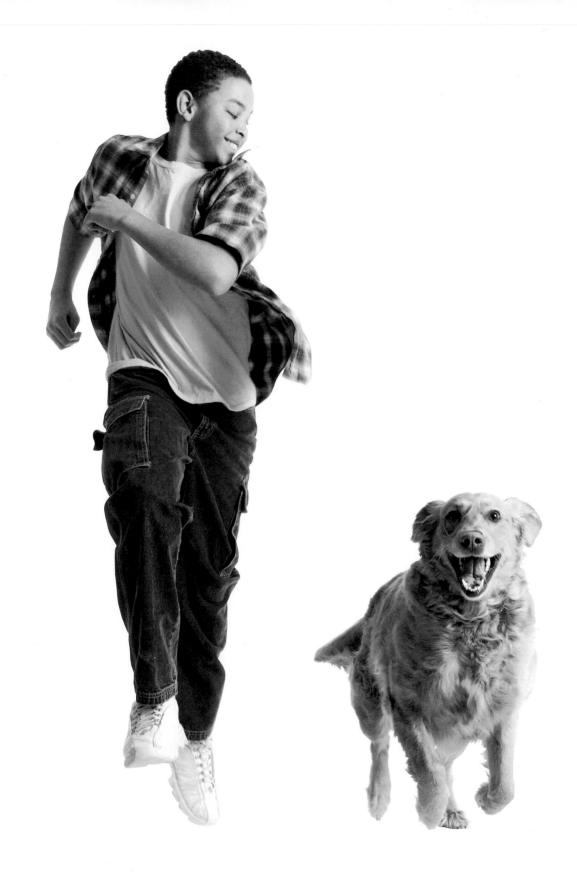

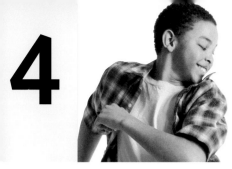

4 getting inspiration

The simple truth is that you are the best inspiration for your children to get active. Researchers now know that children who see their parents, particularly their mother, being active are among the most active themselves.

That doesn't mean that you have to go it alone, especially if you have never been the outdoor or sporty type. Get friends and other members of the extended family involved – arrange picnics and take a ball or a frisbee – things that you'll all find fun.

Spend time with other families who enjoy being active. It's remarkable how your children will gripe if you suggest a family walk, but if you say you're meeting up with friends it's a whole different ball game.

Success breeds success

The other source of inspiration to the previously non-active child is to start seeing good results, and for that to happen you have to give them a head start. Choose an activity that is going to appeal to them, that suits their personality and athletic profile and at which they may shine rather than fail.

There is a sport or activity to suit every child whether they are athletic, non-sporty, sedentary and/or overweight. You must assess whether or not your child is a team player or would be better suited to an individual pastime. Does your child thrive on competition or should you be praising effort, not outcome? There are numerous sports and activities from which to choose and, in order to find what is right for your child, you may have to expose him to a variety of different games.

The important thing is that your child is having fun while he is participating in these activities, and when he finds what suits him he will not only enjoy it but also stick at it.

Which activity?

You've done the hard bit of motivating your family to be more active and to eat healthier food. Now that your child is raring to go, it's time to choose the right activity to maximise her enthusiasm.

We have seen that some children will not want to take part in an organised sport, and would prefer less-structured activity, which is fine. But for those who are now keen to join in an organised sport outside of school, there are some considerations worth taking some time to think about.

- How much time can my child devote to this new sport, either for training or competing?

- How much will it cost to take part and to buy equipment?

- What are the characteristics of the sport – is there physical contact? Is the emphasis on individual or team effort? Will these characteristics suit my child's sporting profile?

- Is my child the right body type (somotype) for this sport? Does it matter?

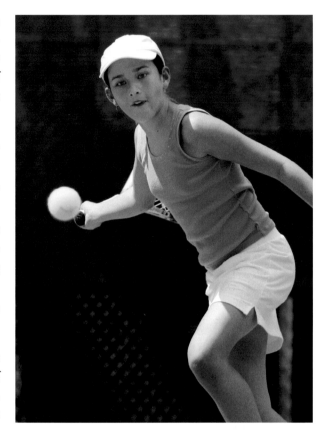

These are questions you might want to consider before giving your child a chance to try out the new sport, but if she is keen I suggest you give it a go, if at all possible. Remember, the emphasis with any new sport is on effort and improvement as much as winning and losing.

Characteristics of the sport

Different sports emphasise different skills. The list on the following page demonstrates which physical and mental skills are promoted by various sports, and from this you can select an activity that may well suit your child's physical aptitude, or that offers experience in the fields in which your child wants to improve.

individual sports	good for
golf	coordination, body control, balance, concentration
cycling	stamina, moderate coordination and concentration
tennis	coordination, body control, speed, stamina, concentration
swimming	strength, stamina
running	speed (sprinting), stamina (distance), moderate concentration
ice skating	flexibility, coordination, body control, concentration
in-line skating/ rollerblading	body control, coordination, moderate flexibility, concentration and stamina
gymnastics	flexibility, coordination, body control, balance, concentration
dancing	flexibility, coordination, body control, concentration
fencing	concentration, body control, agility
skiing	body control, balance, strength,
martial arts	flexibility, body control, concentration
team sports	good for
football	speed, stamina, coordination, concentration, teamwork,
netball/basketball	speed, stamina, coordination, concentration, teamwork, quick thinking
rugby	strength, stamina, coordination, concentration, teamwork, some speed
hockey	strength, coordination, body control, stamina, concentration, teamwork
baseball/rounders	coordination, concentration, teamwork
korfball	speed, stamina, coordination, teamwork, quick thinking

PLAY TO YOUR CHILD'S STRENGTHS

If your child is on the plumper side, then choose sports or activities where weight is an advantage. Rugby and hockey are two sports where weight can be beneficial. Swimming is a good individual activity for overweight kids because they are more buoyant than thinner kids, it doesn't strain joints and they won't get cold as quickly.

In this way, you are setting your child up to do well in something and to feel good about themselves, rather than setting them up to fail.

Know your child's fitness personality

Your child's attitude to taking part in sport and other physical activity will be influenced by his personality, athletic ability and size.

Infants all tend to run around but, as they get older, school-age children tend to fall into three categories:

Non-sporty: Lacks interest in physical activity and often lacks coordination or athletic ability. Will require a lot of motivating.

Casual athlete: Likes taking part in sport but has not got exceptional ability. At risk of getting discouraged in a competitive environment.

Sporty child: Has good coordination, athletic ability and is probably committed to one or more sports or activities. Often highly competitive.

Once you know and understand your child's temperament and fitness profile you are better able to help her to find the activity or sport that she will enjoy.

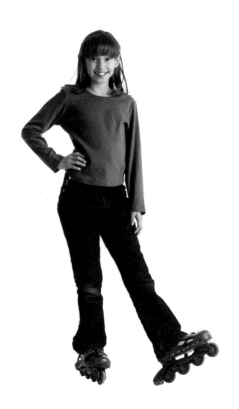

Accepting your body type

We are each born with a specific somotype – or genetically determined body type – and each member of your family will fall into one of three general categories (below). Although there are three distinct body types, as identified by psychologist William H. Sheldon in the 1940s, no one person is completely one body type, but we all have a body type that is predominant.

Your predominant somotype predetermines your physical build. So, it is possible for you to have two lean, long-limbed children and one heavier, more muscular child. What is important is to recognise which somotype each family member is and to explain that, no matter what shape or size, everyone can benefit from a variety of physical activities.

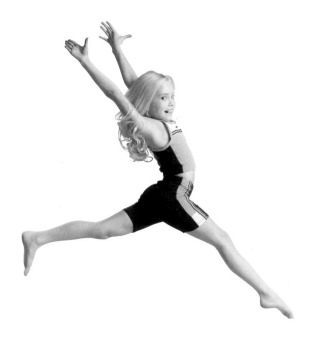

Knowing that we are born with specific body types can help your child to accept the body she has. It can be particularly hard for female siblings if one is lean and rangy and the other considers herself squat and stocky by comparison. It doesn't seem fair that no matter how much exercising she does she may never appear as lean as her sister, and she has a greater tendency to put on weight while the lean one appears to be able to eat anything and not put on an ounce.

It's not fair, but realising that genetics determines body type, skin thickness and where fat tissue is stored may help her to rationalise the difference in their shapes and help her to accept herself as she is. She can then play to her strengths by choosing activities that suit her somotype.

Having said that, if your child has a passion for a sport or pastime, there is no reason why body type should stand in her way. Even short stocky girls can become good netball players if they love the game. And every rugby team needs a nippy, lightweight winger.

Mesomorph

Sheldon described this body type as follows:

- Athletic
- Hard, muscular body
- Rectangular shaped (hourglass shape for women)
- Gains or loses weight easily
- Grows muscle quickly

Best team activities: exercises that require strength and endurance such as rugby, baseball, water polo and ice hockey.

Best individual activities: martial arts, boxing, shot-put, discus, ice skating, sprinting, swimming and gymnastics.

Endomorph

This group has a higher fat-to-muscle ratio. They have a rounded, soft body and women tend to be pear-shaped. Said to have a 'soft look', it can be harder for them to trim and tone through exercise and diet.

The characteristics that Sheldon used to describe an Endomorph body type are as follows:

- Soft body
- Round shaped
- Over-developed digestive system
- Trouble losing weight
- Generally gains muscle easily
- Grows muscle quickly

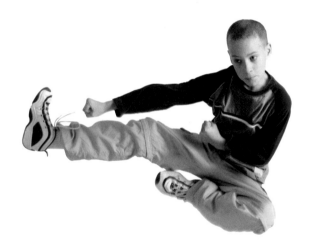

Best activities: middle-distance and moderate-intensity activities are best-suited to this body type. For example swimming, dancing, martial arts, tennis, archery, sailing, golf, hiking, water sports and some field events.

Ectomorph

This is the lanky body type with a narrow pelvic bone. They are typically low in weight and fat and tend to be long and rectangular in shape. These individuals find it hard to put on muscle mass. An Ectomorph body type has difficulty gaining weight and muscle growth takes much longer to achieve and is harder to maintain.

The characteristics that Sheldon used to describe an Ectomorph body type are as follows:

■ Slim

■ Flat chest (girls)

■ Delicate build

■ Tall

■ Lightly muscled

■ Has trouble gaining weight

■ Muscle growth takes longer

Best team activities: football, rugby (winger), basketball, hockey and ice hockey (attacker).

Best individual activities: long-distance running, pole-vaulting, triathlon, cross-country running, skiing and swimming.

Choosing a club

Once you and your child have decided upon a sport or activity, the best way forward is to find a local club. Obviously, word of mouth is hugely important because you cannot beat personal recommendation.

In practice, you often find that children become involved in a club because a classmate or friend is already a member and has encouraged your child to join. This is usually an excellent way to find a club in which your child will be happy and have an existing friend(s) before making new ones. However, if you have any concerns or simply want peace of mind, the tips below still apply.

If you have no personal recommendations or contacts with a club, your local paper or telephone directory will list local clubs. Alternatively, the UK Athletics website (www.athletics.net) has a list of local athletics clubs, and Sport England (www.sportengland.org) and its equivalents in other regions (see Useful contacts on pages 145–50) lists local sports and leisure facilities for your area.

When choosing a sports club, make sure:

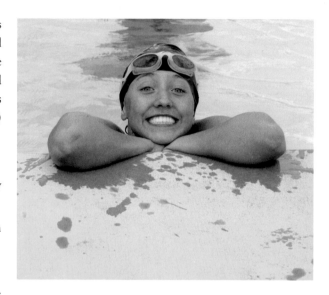

- Any equipment is well-maintained (not necessarily brand new, but in good condition).

- All coaches are fully qualified and have experience in dealing with your child's age group.

- All members of staff have been police checked.

- Security arrangements are in place to stop strangers walking in and interacting with children.

- The facilities are clean and safe.

- The fees are fair and affordable – and find out what sort of annual increases you might expect.

- There is insurance in place in the event that your child is injured.

- The club is accessible so that you can easily drop off and pick up. (Or is there public transport for older children? Is it near enough for her to walk?)

Sport for all

There is no reason why a child with a health problem should not also enjoy the benefits of being more active, albeit that a little more preparation may be required from you. However, it is wise to check with your child's doctor before embarking on a programme of wider activity in case your child's medication needs adjusting. The doctor might also have suggestions on the best ways in which your child can get the most from her activity or sport, given her specific health situation.

There are some chronic conditions, such as asthma and diabetes, that are better suited to some sports than others and some disorders that require special attention to nutritional needs, again diabetes is a good example, but all children with health problems will benefit if they know that they have your support in their sporting endeavours and if you discuss potential problems and obstacles before they embark on specific activities.

tip **BECOME A COACH**
If you would like a greater involvement in your child's sport, you could train as a coach. Sports Coach UK publishes useful fact sheets on becoming a coach and both they and many of the governing bodies for sport, for example the Football Association, the Lawn Tennis Association and UK Athletics, run a series of coaching courses for accreditation.

Why me?

Children like to fit in. Having a chronic health condition can make them feel self-conscious. If your child feels she is drawing attention to herself because she has to use an inhaler before a games lesson, for example, it can be one final obstacle in putting her off doing a sport or activity. However, don't let your child use a health condition as an excuse to be sedentary. All children need to be active, and children with chronic conditions need activity as much as the next child.

A few reassuring words from you that acknowledge how she feels and that offer support could make her feel much better about herself:

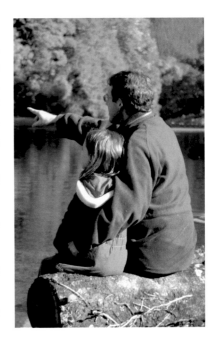

- Talk to her about feeling different, and explain that you understand why she doesn't want to draw attention to herself.

- Make sure she understands why she needs to be responsible about handling her health condition and that it doesn't have to be an obstacle to joining in.

- Give her advice and help on ways to make the management of her condition for sport less conspicuous to others.

- Ensure that teachers and coaching staff are aware of her health needs and ask them to watch for teasing or harassment.

Asthma

Children with asthma often avoid physical activity, either because their parents are protective and don't think it's wise for them to exert themselves, or because they can become uncomfortable and can't keep up with their friends.

Yet, with the right precautions and advice from your doctor, an asthmatic child can actually benefit a great deal from being active because it improves lung capacity and overall fitness. By the same token, being unfit can aggravate asthma symptoms.

The following measures should prove helpful before your child takes up a new sport or activity:

- If your child is on prescribed medication, check with your GP to see if dosages need to be adjusted.

- Cold, dry air can trigger asthma symptoms so she should wear a scarf around her face in these conditions.

fact *Short intense bouts of exercise lasting four to ten minutes are most likely to trigger an asthma attack.*

- If it's very cold she should avoid competing.

- During warm-up time, also practice breathing exercises.

- Dehydration can cause those with breathing difficulties to experience shortness of breath and fatigue. Make sure your child drinks enough, particularly during exercise.

- Inform the instructors and coaches about your child's asthma, so they are on the look out for any signs or symptoms of an impending attack.

- Make sure your child is also aware of what to do in the event of an attack, and make sure she always has her inhaler with her, if appropriate.

Choosing suitable activities

Sports that require short bursts of energy, such as volleyball, rounders, baseball, gymnastics, field events and short-distance track events, could suit asthmatic athletes. With proper supervision, cycling and running can assist in improving cardiorespiratory fitness. Sports that require sustained activity, such as football, can be testing for asthma sufferers.

Swimming is another great activity for kids with asthma because the warm, moist air of the indoor pool makes breathing easier. For the same reason, skiing, ice skating and ice hockey are not recommended since cold air can aggravate the condition.

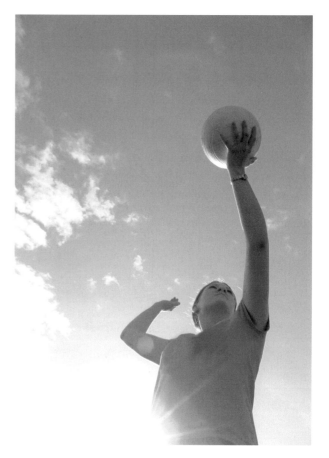

fact *There are a small number of children who have what's known as exercise-induced asthma. Exercise can trigger the following symptoms in these children:*

- *coughing*
- *shortness of breath*
- *chest pain.*

These children can still exercise, on doctor's advice, but they may need to use an inhaler before any physical activity.

Diabetes

Managing diabetes requires a constant balancing of diet, exercise and medication to maintain blood glucose levels as close to normal as possible. Children with both type I (insulin dependent) and type II (non-insulin dependent) diabetes should be encouraged to take part in regular activity.

Exercise is particularly important in keeping blood sugar levels under control and improves the body's response to insulin. Added to which, regular exercise together with a good diet is the best way to maintain a healthy weight, which can reduce the risk of heart disease in adulthood.

The biggest risk from exercise for children with diabetes comes from hypoglycaemia (low blood sugar – see box on page 71). Exercise lowers blood sugar, and since diabetics can have low normal sugar levels this can be a problem if it is not managed.

Once again though, with the right precautions and as long as your child is educated about her condition, the benefits of regular exercise for diabetic children far outweigh the risks. The following list of Dos and Don'ts may help your diabetic child get the most from her physical activities:

- Do talk with your doctor about exercise and how to manage your child's total programme. Some exercises may not be appropriate for her.

- Do make sure teachers, coaches and instructors understand the importance of adhering to your child's meal and snack plan.

- Do try to make sure she exercises every day at the same time. Be as consistent with her exercise as she is with her mealtimes and insulin injections.

- Do exercise soon after eating – when blood sugar levels are at their highest.

- Do get her to test her blood sugar levels before exercising.

- Do ask her to exercise with a friend if possible and be on the lookout for signs of hypoglycaemia.

- Do give her a small snack or fruit juice to eat or drink 15 to 20 minutes before she exercises if her blood sugar levels are not too high. Get her to carry a fast carbohydrate pick-me-up with her when exercising, just in case.

TYPE I AND II DIABETES

There are two principle types of diabetes: type I and type II. With type I, the body is unable to produce any insulin at all, and regular injections of insulin are needed to keep levels of blood sugar as normal as possible. Type 1 is the most common form of diabetes in children: 90–95 per cent of under 16s with diabetes have this type.

However, type II diabetes, previously known as adult-onset diabetes, is on the increase in children. It is rarely seen in people who are not overweight, and scientists predict that as the obesity epidemic spreads so the number of children who develop type II diabetes will continue to grow.

Those with type II diabetes can make insulin, but the body does not respond to it normally so oral medication and/or injections may be needed.

Diabetes increases the risk of developing heart disease, strokes and kidney failure in later life.

- Don't inject insulin into a part of the body that's being exercised. It will be absorbed faster there.

- Don't exercise when insulin is working at peak action. If she must, she should eat before she exercises.

- Do make sure adults supervising your child during sports or activities know what to do in case of an emergency.

- Do get her to carry or wear medical identification giving the necessary emergency information.

Choosing suitable activities

A child with diabetes can have a go at any sport as long as she bears in mind the advice about monitoring blood sugar and follows the above precautions. If she has been newly diagnosed, it is best to pick a sport that is 'continuous' such as cycling, swimming or walking/hiking since it is easier to calculate and monitor how much energy is being expended and therefore how much glucose will be used.

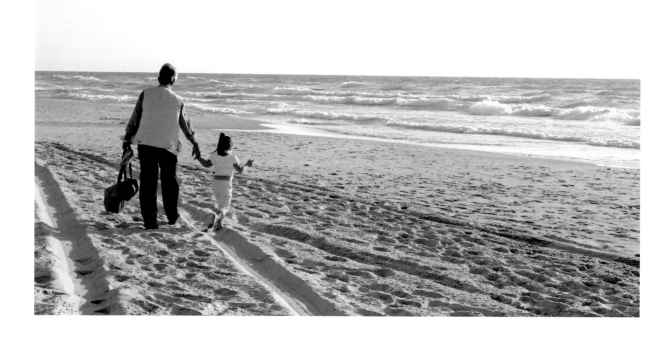

WHAT IS HYPOGLYCAEMIA?

If your child's blood sugar levels drop too low, it is known as hypoglycaemia or 'hypo'. This can be caused by a variety of different reasons, but it's mainly when they have had:

- too much insulin

- not enough food

- an excessive amount of exercise

- a delayed meal

- stress

- time in hot weather.

It is important that you and your child remember how she feels when she is having a hypo and make sure that your child, family and friends, teachers and coaches know what to look for if it happens again. Common symptoms include:

- hunger

- shaking/wobbly legs

- butterflies in the tummy

- sweating

- headache

- faintness

- dizziness

- blurred vision.

If a hypo is not treated, your child could become confused, sleepy or even lose consciousness.

The best way to treat a hypo is to give your child sugar or food containing sugar straight away followed by a sandwich or carbohydrate-rich snack. That's why it is so important for kids with diabetes to carry an emergency snack. They should also carry ID saying they have diabetes and explaining what to do in case of an emergency. In extreme cases, your child may need to be given an injection of a medication that raises blood sugar levels.

ADHD

Given that many parents of children with Attention Deficit Hyperactivity Disorder (ADHD) report that they have boundless energy, you might be forgiven for assuming that sport comes naturally to these children. And it is true that, with the right encouragement and understanding from instructors, sport can help a child with ADHD gain more control over her movement and improve her social skills.

Yet, children with ADHD also face problems in sport because they can find it hard to follow instruction, they may take unnecessary risks not only with

fact *The last 30 years has seen a threefold increase in the number of cases of childhood diabetes. In England and Wales 17 children per 100,000 develop diabetes each year. In Scotland the figure is 25 per 100,000.*

themselves but also with other participants, and they may have difficulty concentrating for a full match or session.

That is not to say that, in the right conditions, sport cannot be beneficial to a child with ADHD. It can be a very positive channel for excess energy and the sense of achievement when such a child succeeds in a sport can work wonders for her self-esteem. Moreover, the ability to be a team player learned through sport can help your child feel more confident and make friends more easily.

As parents, you can help to make sport and activity a positive experience for your ADHD child by:

- ensuring that the coach/instructor understands your child's particular characteristics and needs.

- attending training and helping to supervise your child, especially where equipment is involved.

- helping your child to understand the need to wait her turn, to listen to instructions and to be part of the team.

- if your child takes medication, checking with your GP to find out whether the dosage needs to be adjusted.

Choosing suitable activities

All sports are good, as they will improve body awareness. However, individual sports such as tennis, swimming, dancing and martial arts can be good for a child with ADHD as she is likely to get more personal tuition from a coach than in a team sport.

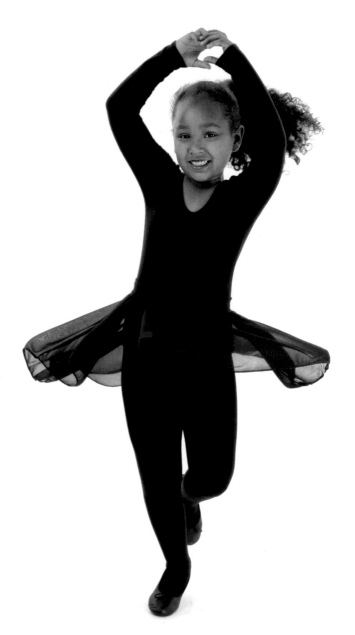

SPECIAL NEEDS

Physical activity benefits children with disabilities but they often have a tough time getting started. With the best of intentions, parents of children with health problems or disabilities may fear that their child could be injured by sports or exercise or that it may worsen her condition, and so they do not encourage participation.

Yet, in most cases – and obviously with the permission of her medical specialists – a child with disabilities can gain huge satisfaction and benefit from being active, not least because it can be a boost to her self-esteem as she experiences a sense of accomplishment and possibly the taste of winning.

In recent years, huge strides have been made in the design and provision of sports equipment for children with disabilities. From hand-crank tricycles to snow skis, sports wheelchairs to special horse-riding saddles, the variety of choice is so much wider now.

Depending on the condition involved (hearing and visual impairment, birth defect such as cerebral palsy, developmental disabilities, heart problems, brain or spinal cord injuries, muscular dystrophy, and seizure disorders) benefits from physical activity can include:

- muscle strengthening
- greater joint mobility
- improved balance and coordination.

You can encourage your child with special needs to be physically active by:

- Researching local sports groups such as wheelchair basketball leagues, adapted horse riding and tennis leagues in your local area.

- Help your child to set his own personal goals – and not to strive for somebody else's.

- Praise her efforts and remark on achievements – even if they appear small or progress seems painfully slow.

- If she finds a sport she loves, help her to get the most from it and to continue by providing the necessary adaptive sports equipment.

Parent power

Once you start enquiring about school and local sports/activities, there may be more going on in your area than you suspect. You may be amazed at what's available in terms of local initiatives for both healthy eating and getting kids active.

But – and here we go again, because it's a big but – if you find there is a dearth of grass-roots activity locally then it might be down to you (and other interested parents) to make things happen. Not that I'm suggesting you stride into your child's school demanding healthier school dinners and more hours devoted to PE, but what I am saying is that you should not underestimate the influence of parent power.

What can you do?

Firstly, you can look at the areas that affect your child. Are you happy with the quality of food served in your child's school? Is there a junior football team locally for your son's age group? If there are gaps in the provision you can do something about it – either by applying pressure or by actively setting something up.

For example, you could get together with other concerned parents and approach the school about a change in policy. Also get the Parents and Teachers Association (PTA) on board to apply pressure. If the school still won't budge, bring school governors and the local authority into the equation. If enough people show that they are concerned about the health of our children then things will change for the better. And, although it may seem like a small victory on a modest local scale, if every concerned parent takes action then it becomes a change of attitude on a national scale, and so on.

Similarly, if your daughter and her friends are keen to play netball in a league, and there is no club locally, then why not set one up? Ask other parents to be involved and seek advice from the local league on what is required.

There are obviously regulations to satisfy in terms of police checking etc. before you can work with young people, but there's plenty of advice on these issues. Your first port of call for information on this front would be The Child Protection in Sport Unit (see Useful contacts on pages 145–50). And, if funding is an issue, there are grants and courses available for interested parents: Sports Coach UK produces some useful fact sheets on becoming a coach.

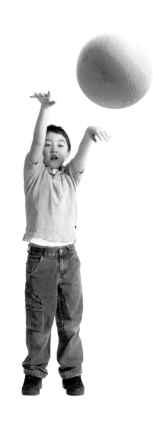

SCHOOL DINNERS

OK, admittedly, he's a celebrity but Jamie Oliver's School Dinners campaign just goes to prove what can be done if enough people care. He delivered a petition to Prime Minister Tony Blair with 271,677 signatures on it in March 2005. As a result, the Government pledged an extra £280 million to improve school meals.

Get inspired

Still don't believe that you can make a difference? Take a look at the following initiatives already in place that you can call upon to support you, your child and your healthy living aspirations, and which might just give you the inspiration and the boost you need to get going.

Healthy eating initiatives

■ **The Food Dude Healthy Eating Programme** – This programme has been developed by psychologists at the University of Wales, Bangor, and is an initiative to encourage children to improve their diets and, specifically, to eat more fruit and vegetables. It is designed for use in primary schools and parents/schools who have used the programme report outstanding and, more importantly, long lasting results. For example, a school in Salford reported that consumption of fruit at lunchtime was up by 154 per cent and vegetable consumption had risen by a whopping 300 per cent.

The programme uses videos featuring hero figures called – yes, you guessed it – the 'Food Dudes' who are cool but who like fruit and vegetables, and small rewards (e.g. stickers, notebooks, pencils) to ensure that the children begin to taste new foods.

To find out more about introducing the Food Dude Programme in your child's school, visit www.fooddudes.co.uk.

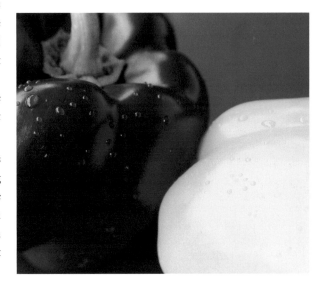

■ **Jamie Oliver's Feed Me Better campaign** also has School Starter Packs but, due to overwhelming popularity, these have sold out. Not to worry because you can still download sample pages from www.feedmebetter.com and there should be enough information in these pages for a school to implement the initiative.

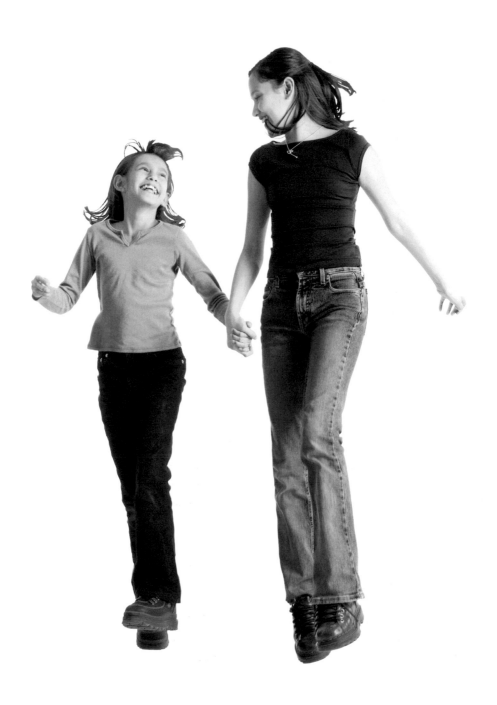

■ In the same way, Channel 4's **School Dinner's** campaign, again involving Jamie Oliver, offers a downloadable action pack specifically for parents as well as a review of the campaign's success. Go to http://www.channel4.com/life/microsites/J/jamies_school_dinners/index.html.

Getting active initiatives

■ The **Primary Playgrounds 4 Sports Scheme** allows schools to invest in simple playground markings at minimal outlay to promote structured play for children. A partnership was formed by The Football Foundation, The Youth Sports Trust, The Football Association, The Lawn Tennis Association, The Rugby Football Union and the England and Wales Cricket Board to help increase the levels of physical activity in the playground and to offer children a wider choice of activity.

A full playground resource pack provides a series of steps to support schools with the development, redesign and improvement of their playground – from involving the children to training key staff and monitoring the new playground's impact. It is available together with a Primary Playgrounds 4 Sport application form from http://www.footballfoundation.org.uk/seeking-funding/capital-projects/primary-playgrounds-4-sports-initiative.

■ Each year, more than a million children across the UK develop their sports skills by taking part in **athletics schemes** (organised by UK Athletics and sponsored by Norwich Union). These schemes offer something for all ages and abilities and give children an opportunity to try events that they would not normally have a chance to sample such as pole-vaulting, discus and javelin. For details, visit www.ukathletics.net.

■ David Beckham famously benefited from the Bobby Charlton Soccer School and Sports Academy (which still offers summer schools, residential courses and provides many courses for schools and junior clubs from around the UK and into Europe) and, as testament to his gratitude, he has now set up **The David Beckham Football Academy**. Similarly, the DBFA offers soccer camps, schools education programmes and coach education programmes. For further details on both Academies, see Useful contacts on pages 145–50.

- **The Lawn Tennis Association** is helping to increase the accessibility of tennis across Great Britain. They provide support in the development of programmes, coach education and advice as well as financial support. The support provided is primarily through funding pay and play facilities and through funding the kick-starting of affordable structured tennis programmes on park courts. (See Useful contacts on pages 145–50).

These are just a few of the many schemes and initiatives to help support and develop an interest in sport at junior levels. If your child is interested in a sport that is not mentioned in the above list, and there is not a provision locally, then it is worth contacting the governing body for the game/sport to find out whether there are resources and schemes available that might benefit your neighbourhood or local school.

fact

- In 2004 a Mori poll revealed that almost 50 per cent of schools did not organise a competitive school sports day.
- Ofsted report that one in five British schools have inadequate sports facilities.
- About 50 per cent of schoolchildren do not receive 2 hours of physical education each week.

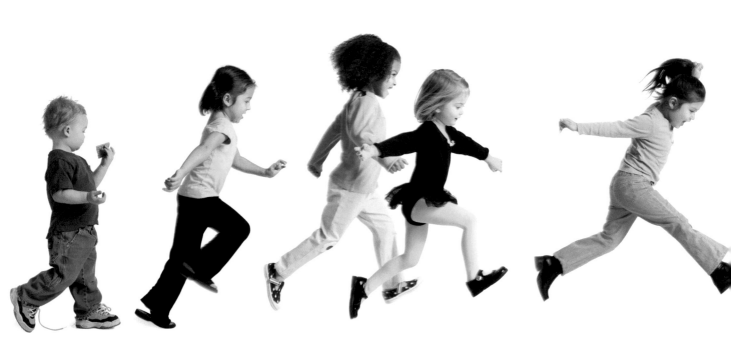

OVERCOMING BARRIERS

Wheel Power, the national charity for British Wheelchair Sport, has details on a whole host of initiatives and schemes to provide opportunities for disabled children to enjoy the enormous benefits of taking part in sport. For details of The Norwich Union Junior Heroes sports activity camps and the Junior Games held at the Stoke Mandeville stadium (the national disabled sports centre) visit www.wheelpower.org.uk.

tip *Most Premiership football clubs run Football in the Community schemes to encourage young talent at grassroots. They provide coaches to run training sessions at local schools. So, if you have a club near you it could be worth approaching them through your child's school.*

fact

If you want your child to be more active and to join a club but sport isn't her bag, then a youth group or guides/scouts could prove a better route (see Useful Contacts). She will get social activities as well as an opportunity to take part in all sorts of indoor/outdoor pursuits.

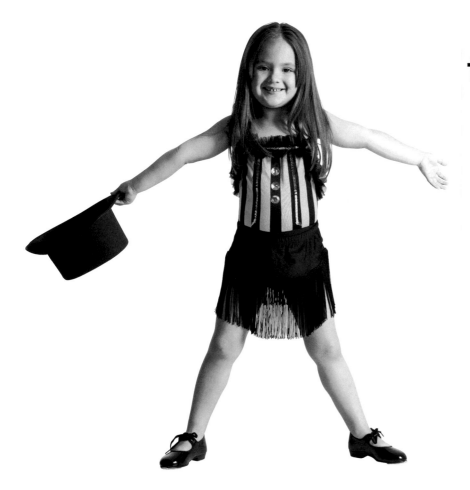

Q&A

Question: How will I know if my child has exercise-induced asthma?

Answer: If your child experiences shortness of breath, fatigue or a dry cough after exercise, you should visit your doctor who can perform a simple test to confirm (or otherwise) exercise-induced asthma. The GP will measure your child's breathing volume while she is at rest. Then she will perform about 10 minutes of exercise (often on a stationary bicycle) after which her lung volume will be measured again at five, ten and fifteen minute intervals. If there is a drop in volume of more than 10 per cent exercise-induced asthma is the likely cause.

Question: My daughter's school has no playing fields and puts very little emphasis on sport. Is this common?

Answer: According to a recent Government audit, in 1992 there were 78,000 school playing fields on 26,00 sites in England, but by 2005 this figure had fallen to 44,000 playing fields on 21,000 sites. In the last 13 years nearly half of school playing fields have been sold off, so it is no surprise that less than two-thirds of school pupils receive the Government's target of 2 hours or more physical education each week. Sadly, your child's school is not unusual.

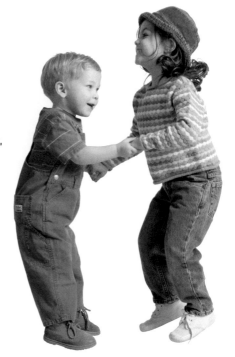

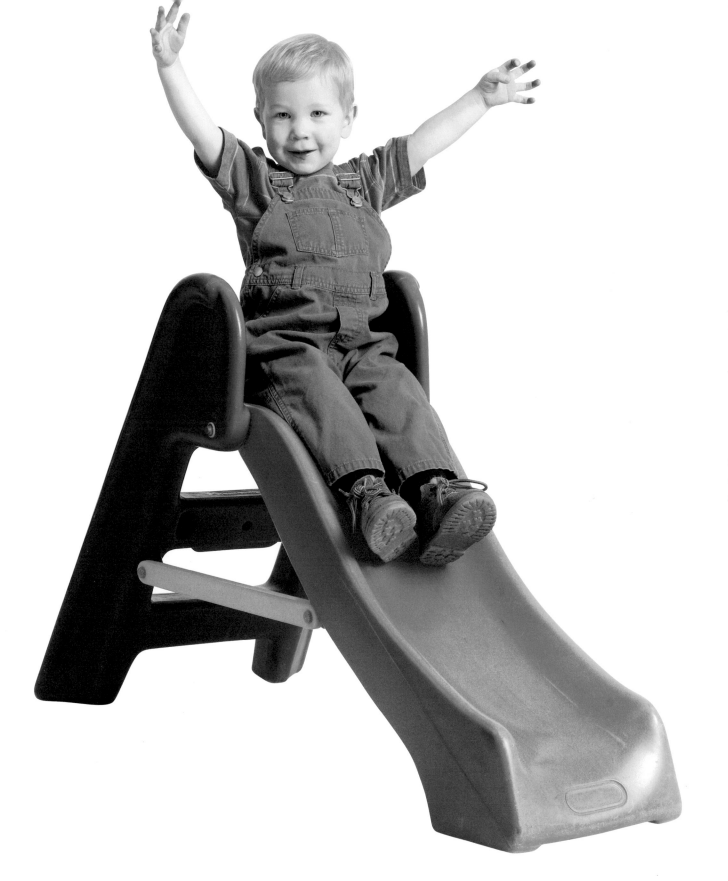

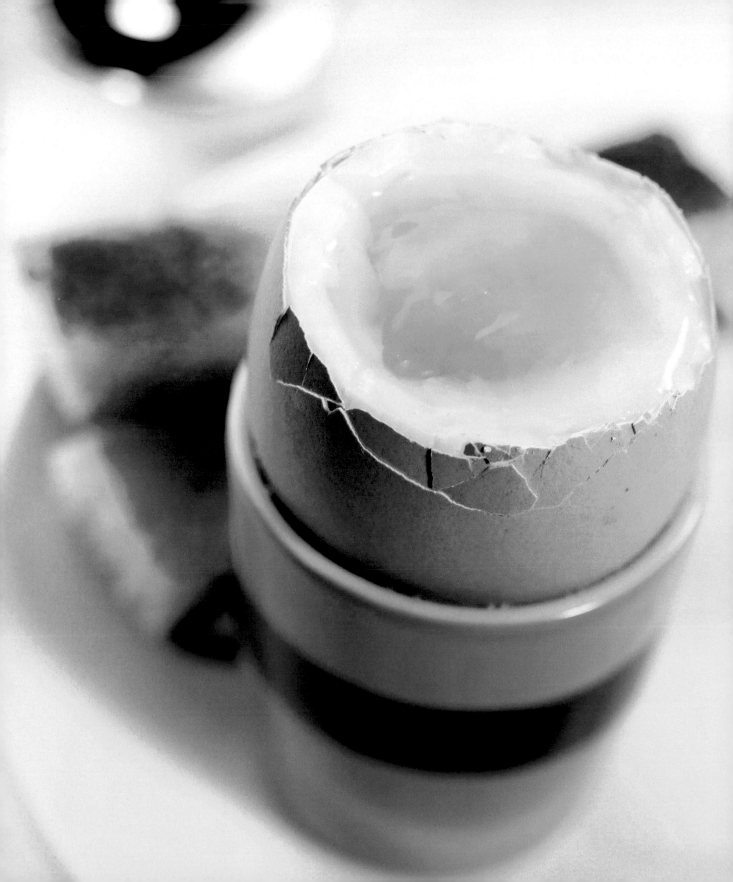

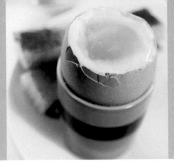

5 good food attitude

Getting you and your children more active is the main aim of this book, but it would be pointless to get everyone on the move and not to address the problem of what you eat. A balanced diet is an integral part of a healthier lifestyle and it is also essential if you and your family are to have the energy for all the extra activity that you are planning.

Unfortunately, I recognise that it's not easy to get the balance right between the number of calories consumed and the amount of energy expended through physical activity. For many families, the daily schedule is so jammed full that finding the time to prepare and eat balanced meals together and to exercise is problematic.

Nonetheless, we have seen in the previous chapter how you can build extra activity into your busy agenda, and now we will look at simple ways to make sure that your children are eating the right foods too.

Food revolution

After a long day at school and work, many families find preparing and waiting for a healthy meal just too much of a challenge. Everyone's hungry and convenience foods seem the obvious answer.

However, a typical fast-food meal contains a lot of calories for a small amount of food, a characteristic that is known as 'energy dense' in nutritional circles. The Medical Research Council shows that a fast-food meal has more than one and a half times the calories of a similar-sized portion of a traditional British home-cooked meal.

In addition, we eat out more frequently than ever before and restaurant foods, particularly fast-food restaurants, are laden with far more calories than home-cooked meals. And it is not just what your kids are eating but how much. Portion sizes have increased drastically over the past 20 years, with some fast-food chains actively encouraging children to super-size their meals. In some cases, fast-food portions are up to six times the size that was consumed in 1955.

If you are concerned that your child is eating too much convenience or fast food, or that she grazes on chocolate bars, sweets or salty snacks too often, or

> **fact** In the 1960s it took on average about two and a half hours to prepare an evening meal; with the advent of convenience foods, it now takes about 15 minutes.

simply that television advertising holds too much sway over her tastes, then it is time to make a change.

The first step is to make sure that your child understands the link between a healthy diet together with regular exercise and her emotional and physical well-being. Without doubt, a diet high in fat and sugar may seem appetising to the young (and possibly to you also) but too much of it will leave your child feeling lethargic and depressed and, in many cases, overweight.

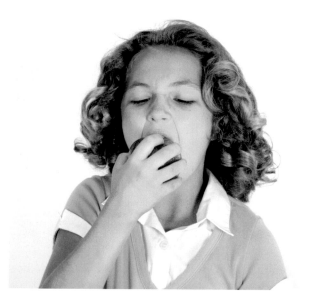

Shaping your child's eating habits in early life will set her on the right path for a lifetime of good nutrition and good health. If you let her get into bad habits now, in all probability, it will only get worse as she gets older.

Remember, healthy eating doesn't have to mean boring meals. It's up to you to make nutritious foods appealing and fun for your family and to help them to form a good food attitude.

What is a healthy diet?

Although each family's diet will vary depending on tradition, culture and personal taste there are a few basic guidelines that apply to us all.

Children need to eat the right food to stay healthy, not just now but in the future. A nutritious diet will:

- help them to grow
- keep them healthy, fit and looking well
- fend off illness
- give them energy
- help them to concentrate and do better in school.

To provide your child with the nutrients she needs, you should always offer a wide variety of foods. It is obviously easier if you have done this since their earliest age but it is never too late to start introducing more variety into your child's diet.

fact *In 2005 in the USA, 12.2 million visits to big brand food websites were made by children younger than 11.*

Eighty-five per cent of US food companies target children on websites. They are able to circumvent strict rules on marketing to children because information on websites is regarded as editorial material, not advertising.

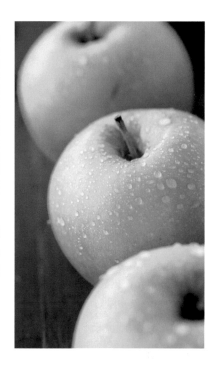

If you serve foods from each of the seven food groups (based on the World Health Organisation nutritional recommendations), you stand a greater chance of meeting their daily nutritional requirements. The seven food groups are:

- grains and potatoes

- dairy products

- meat and other protein-rich foods

- fruit

- vegetables

- healthy fats and oils

- fatty and sugary foods.

How much?

Unfortunately, there is no simple answer to this question. The truth is that what your child needs from her diet changes as she ages. As an infant she needs almost half of her daily calories from fat, but by the time she is at primary school she only needs about one-third from fat and the majority from carbohydrates.

If you ensure that none of the food groups are excluded totally from your child's diet, and you try to roughly follow the ratio of portions from each group as outlined on the following page, you should offer a balanced, nutritious diet.

- **Grains and potatoes**: These include bread, pasta, noodles, cereals, rice, crackers, potatoes, parsnips and yams. Target: 4–6 portions per day.

- **Fruit and vegetables**: The government's five-a-day initiative may sound like a lot – and it's woefully true that only one in five children hits this target – but if your child has an apple and some cucumber chunks in her packed lunch and you serve two vegetables at the evening meal together with a glass of fruit juice, that's the target met. Not so bad, after all. Target: 5–9 portions per day.

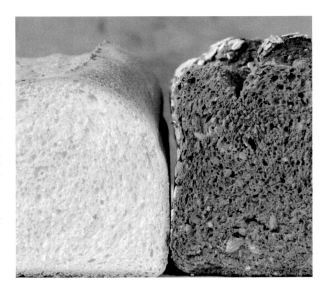

- **Dairy products:** These include milk, cheese, yoghurt and fromage frais. Target: 2–4 portions per day.

- **Meat and other protein-rich foods**: Lean meat, chicken, turkey, fish, eggs, soya, quorn, tofu, beans, lentils and nuts. Target: 2–4 portions per day.

- **Healthy fats and oils**: For example, nuts (walnuts, Brazils, cashews, pine nuts, almonds, pecans) and seeds (sesame, sunflower, pumpkin), seed oils (rapeseed and sunflower), nut oils (olive oil) and oily fish* (sardines, mackerel, pilchards). Target: 1–2 portions per day. (*Once or twice a week is enough for children due to high content of essential fats.)

- **Fatty and sugary foods**: Examples include cakes, biscuits, sweets, fizzy drinks, chocolate, crisps and other snacks. Target: Although official recommendations allow up to one portion per day, it is suggested that you offer this food group only in moderation – once a week is probably a better target.

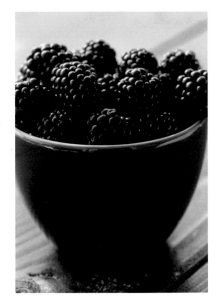

Rainbow eating

Different coloured fruit and vegetables provide different vitamins, minerals and healthy phytochemicals, so try to get your child to eat a rainbow of different coloured fruit and vegetables throughout the week.

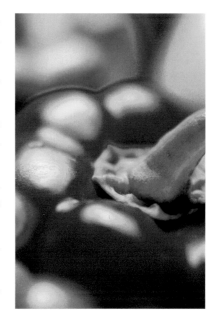

- **Red** fruit and vegetables are rich in immune-boosting vitamin C. Red peppers contain lutein for healthy eyes; tomatoes and watermelon contain lycopene – an antioxidant that helps protect cells.

- **Yellow** fruits such as bananas offer zinc and potassium, which help to regulate fluid balance.

- **Orange** fruit and vegetables are rich in betacarotene, which is a good source of vitamin A and helps boost the immune system and promotes eye and skin health. They also contain carotenoids and bioflavonoids.

- **White** vegetables such as onions and garlic have natural antibacterial and anti-inflammatory properties. They also provide allicins, which boost the immune system.

- **Green** leafy vegetables are rich in vitamins A and C, fibre and nutrients such as calcium and folate. Most green vegetables are also a good source of iron.

- **Blue and purple** fruits such as blueberries and plums contain anthocyanins, which neutralise harmful free radicals that damage cells.

WEASEL WORDS

Packaging claims such as 'healthy', 'fresh', 'natural', 'farmhouse', 'wholesome' or 'nutritious' aim to reassure the consumer about a food's origins and health credentials but these should be treated with caution. None of these words are defined by law and are often meaningless. Similarly terms such as 'lite' or 'light' have no legal definition and may be found on high-calorie products. You have been warned – it pays to read the small print on the label.

RECOMMENDED DAILY ALLOWANCES

You have probably seen RDA levels on food packaging. These are the government's Recommended Daily Allowances (RDAs) and they give useful guidance on the right amount of nutrients needed per serving size and per gram of food each day. However, this system can be difficult to monitor and to adhere to religiously. Sometimes a better rule of thumb is to make sure that your child is getting a diet full of variety, freshness and colour.

tip **GETTING YOUR KIDS TO EAT MORE FRUIT AND VEG**

- *Try freezing grapes for a cool treat, or alternate chunks of banana, cherry and grape on a wooden skewer and place in the freezer to make delicious and healthy kebabs.*
- *Rinse and cut oranges into quarters with the peel on to make them easier to eat. Then make the skins into 'false teeth' afterwards (cut the skin down the middle and then across – like melon boats – but leaving a border. Then insert between lips and teeth, pith-side out and cause a laugh with your funky false teeth!)*
- *Cut apples into eight slices for easy eating and put washed grapes in a handy little bunch in the fridge at kid eye-level.*
- *Take your child to a 'pick your own' fruit farm – you'll be amazed how much she wolfs down while picking.*
- *Buy kid-friendly sized vegetables such as baby sweet corn, peeled baby carrots, baby courgettes and new potatoes.*
- *Instead of serving a pile of vegetables on your child's plate thread them on a skewer to add interest.*

Cutting back on sugary and high-fat foods

Rather than forbidding high-fat or high-sugar foods and sweets outright, it is an easier and often more successful option to limit the supply of these 'treats' and to offer healthier alternatives in their place.

The best way to bolster your resolve is to make sure you don't have these 'temptation' foods in your home. This results in a win:win situation. Firstly, if your child doesn't see biscuits, sweets and cakes in the cupboard she is less inclined to ask for them or crave them. Secondly, if she does ask for such foods, you can draw the pestering to a close by legitimately saying, 'We don't have that in the house. So would you like an apple or some raisins?'

By offering a variety of alternative healthy options, your child will be lulled into feeling that she has a choice and therefore a degree of control, albeit that she can't have her original 'temptation' food.

If you are going to keep these 'temptation' foods in the house then at least buy them in smaller amounts and sizes. So, if you allow your child a treat, offer an individually-wrapped, fun-size chocolate bar rather than a full-size, or opt for a small packet of crisps rather than letting her dip into a family-size bag.

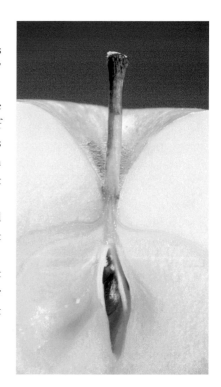

Other measures to cut down on high-sugar and high-fat foods include:

- Keep sweets and chocolates to a specific time once a week – perhaps a Saturday or Sunday afternoon. If she is given sweets in the interim, she can put them away until the prescribed 'treat' time.

- Discourage your child's sweet tooth by limiting sweet foods, even those that are artificially sweetened.

- When home cooking, add less sugar than the recipe recommends.

- Check labels for hidden sugars. For example, a small can of pasta shapes contains 2 teaspoons of sugar and a fruit winder or small fruit yoghurt contains 3 teaspoons.

tip *When kids get home from school, they will often say that they're starving and reach for the first high-energy snack they can find. You can pre-empt this by having a platter of fruit chunks for each of them or some cheese and crackers ready and waiting. For older kids, you can always fall back on wholemeal toast and peanut butter or a bowl of wholegrain breakfast cereal to fill them up.*

fact **More weasel words**
'No added sugar' on the label does not mean that the product contains no sugar. It may have a high natural sugar content from other ingredients such as fruit juice.
As a rule of thumb, the Food Standards Agency suggests that foods with more than 10 g of sugar per 100 g are high and less than 2 g per 100 g are low.

tip *Dilution is a good strategy when it comes to snacks. If your child loves crisps mix a few in a small bag with other healthier snack foods, such as mini rice cakes, pretzels and peanuts.*

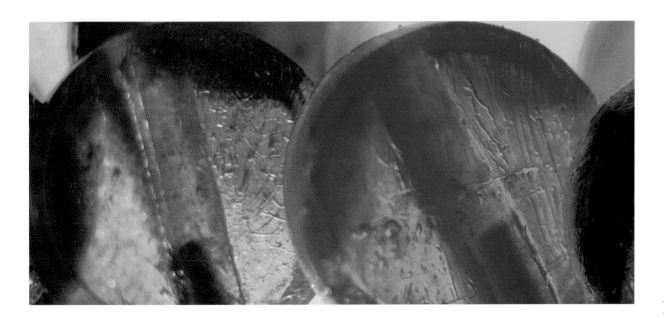

SHOULD KIDS EAT A LOW-FAT DIET?

Children should not be put on restrictive diets. Despite all the bad press, fat and cholesterol play an important role in brain development in young children, so fat intake should never be restricted in under two-year-olds.

Having said that, it's true that most British kids eat too much fat so, from the age of two, you should be aiming for your child's fat intake to provide about 30 per cent of her total calorie intake. To achieve this, you can:

- Choose cooking methods that allow fat to drip away such as grilling or roasting on a rack. Avoid frying where possible.

- Offer naturally low-fat foods such as lean meats, whole grains, fruit and vegetables, and choose low-fat dairy products.

- From two years old, you can start giving your toddler semi-skimmed milk. Fully skimmed milk isn't suitable as a main drink until they're five years old, because it doesn't contain enough calories for a growing child.

- Restrict fat-laden snacks and fast foods. A bag of crisps has 10 g of fat and a chicken nugget from a typical fast-food chain contains nearly 60 per cent fat.

- Cut back on mayonnaise, butter and margarine.

tip *Ingredients are listed in diminishing order of quantity. So the product contains the first ingredient in the greatest quantity, and so on. Beware of foods or drinks that list: sugar, sucrose, dextrose, glucose syrup or high-fructose corn syrup in the top three ingredients.*

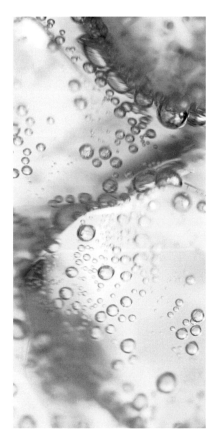

Can the can

Increased consumption of fizzy drinks and fruit squashes – which contain more sugar than any other item in most children's diet – is causing particular concern among health experts.

In a study published in the journal *Pediatrics*, researchers from The Children's Hospital Boston, USA, followed 103 teenagers for 6 months. Their results showed that drinking a single 330 ml can of sugar-sweetened drink each day translated to a 0.5 kg weight gain every 3 to 4 weeks. Hence, teenagers who consume a can of sugary drink a day are likely to be up to 6.4 kg heavier after a year than those drinking unsweetened versions.

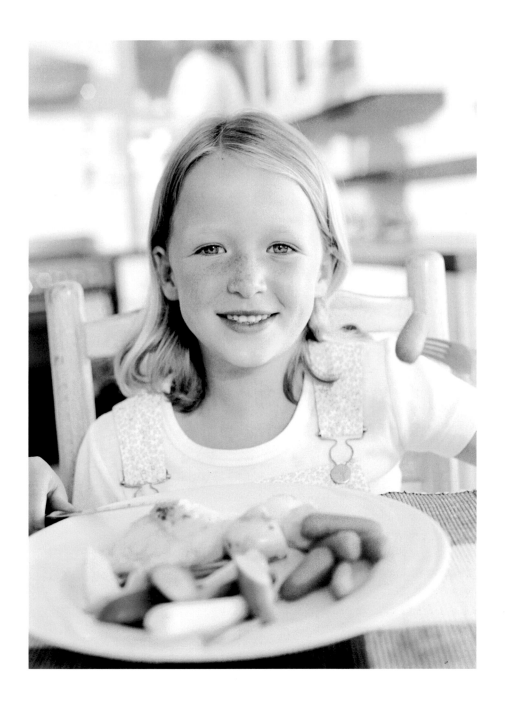

The facts speak for themselves. Your child's consumption of canned and bottled soft drinks should be severely curbed, both for their general health and for the sake of their teeth in particular. Healthier options are:

■ water

■ semi-skimmed milk

■ milkshakes with fresh fruit (no added sugar)

■ 100 per cent fruit juice (although not to excess because calories from the natural sugars in fruit juice can soon add up). This can be diluted with water to much better effect.

Helping kids to eat healthily

It's all well and good to know what your child should be eating, but actually persuading them to change their eating habits and to ditch the bad stuff for the good can be easier said than done.

However, the following tricks and tips are collected from experts and parents alike and have been proven to work in the fight against bad eating habits.

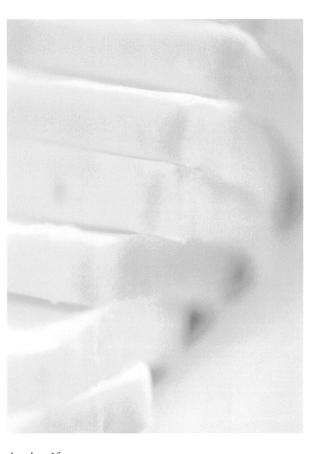

Be realistic

It's very easy to allow food to become the cause of family battles. If you get worked up when your child rejects new foods or healthier options, she'll pick up on these negative feelings and will either become stressed herself or will instinctively know how to 'push your buttons' on food issues. Stay relaxed and don't take a rejection of food as a rejection of you or a personal slight on your parenting skills. Just persevere and recognise that sometimes it will work well and sometimes it won't.

tip *Eating a small piece of cheese, which is alkali, after a sugary or acidic drink or snack helps counteract the harmful effects of sugar and fruit acids on the teeth.*

Let them choose

Rather than piling food on to individual plates, put food out in serving bowls and allow your kids to help themselves – with the proviso that they have at least two of the three vegetables on offer. They're more likely to eat what they put on their own plates rather than what you serve up.

Make meals a social occasion

Eating the same food as your children, at the same time, is a great way to model good habits and to make mealtimes fun.

Kids in the kitchen

Encourage children to help prepare new foods. According to the Food Standards Agency (FSA) research suggests they will be more likely to try new foods if they've had a hand in their preparation.

Make healthy food appealing

You can jazz up a plain apple or boring meat and two veg to make it look attractive and exciting. Why not offer apple slices with a yoghurt dip or sprinkle some grated cheese over the top of broccoli or cauliflower? Sometimes texture is important to kids, so if they prefer their vegetables crispy and crunchy then let them eat them raw as crudités – either on their own or with hummus, salsa or a yoghurt dip.

Keep it accessible

If you have fruit on display in a fruit bowl, your child is more likely to pick a piece when she is feeling peckish.

Get seasonal

Introduce new fruits and vegetables as they come into season. Summer fruits, such as strawberries, nectarines, peaches and raspberries, and vegetables, such as courgettes and tomatoes, could be exchanged for blackberries, blueberries and plums in the autumn and these then change to grapes and clementines, parsnips and Brussels sprouts in the winter.

Grow your own

To reinforce the seasonal theme, you could always have a crack at growing your own. You don't need a great deal

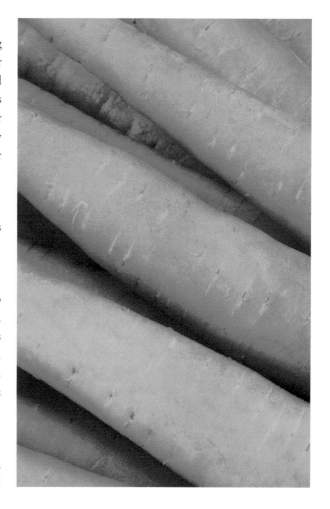

of space to make a small vegetable patch or you can even use growbags on patios. The most successful varieties in our experience (when the dog doesn't dig them up!) are potatoes, tomatoes, courgettes, leeks and runner beans.

A little is better than nothing

If your child only likes one or two vegetables, it's not the end of the world. Keep serving these and occasionally try her with a new vegetable until she extends her repertoire.

Trick them, if necessary

If your child still adamantly refuses anything that resembles a fresh vegetable, then disguise them in food – or trick your child into eating them. All-in-one dishes such as bolognese sauce, shepherd's pie, hot pot and chilli are all ideal for disguising finely chopped vegetables such as peppers, sweetcorn, carrots and onions. Smooth soups are another great way of disguising fresh, healthy ingredients and kids love them.

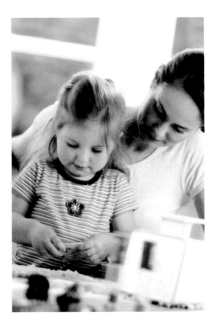

SIX OF THE BEST: HEALTHY EATING TIPS FOR PARENTS

- **Be a role model**. Where healthy eating is concerned, 'do as I do' is definitely the order of the day. If they see you eating healthily, they're most likely to copy.

- **Give them a chance**. Where is it written that all kids prefer junk food to nutritious meals? Parents and restaurateurs just assume it: hence the proliferation of unimaginative kiddie menus offering only nuggets, fish fingers and burgers. In fact, the 4Children survey in 2006 showed that eight out of ten children say they like vegetables and fruit. Let your kids sample new tastes and food experiences, and they may surprise you.

- **Supply and demand**. Remember, you decide which foods to buy and when to serve them, so dump the junk.

- **Let them choose**. If you're supplying only good food, then there's no harm in letting your kids decide which bits they eat, and how much. The 'clean plate brigade' has had its day – encourage them to try everything, but allow them to stop eating when they've had enough.

- **Rewards**. Don't confuse food with love. There are better ways to reward your kids and to show them that you love them than giving them sweets as treats.

- **Catch them early**. Children's food preferences are formed early in life, so the sooner you offer a variety of foods the better.

Hunger vs. cravings

There is a difference between feeling hungry and craving something to eat, but your child may not be able to tell the difference. You can help him recognise when he actually needs food (hunger) or if he is acting on internal emotions, habit or an external stimulus (craving).

Cravings can occur at any time, not necessarily when your child is hungry. If she eats because he craves something, it is one of the quickest and easiest ways to consume too many calories and, for many kids, to gain weight.

Common stimuli for kids' cravings are:

- Seeing food that they like – and wanting it.
- Seeing food advertised on the TV or in a magazine.
- Someone offering them food and, even though they're not hungry, they are not able to say no.
- Smelling food as they pass a bakery or take-away shop.
- Seeing sweets at the supermarket checkout and not wanting to pass by empty-handed.
- Eating while watching a film/DVD/TV/computer game because they're in the habit of doing so.
- Having a dessert after a large meal because it's customary.
- Eating supper before going to bed because they always have.

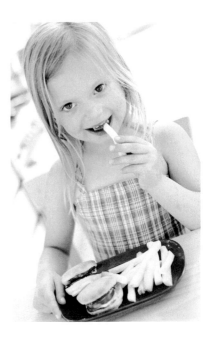

Once you've identified if your child eats out of craving rather than hunger, and it's highly likely that this is the case, then try to train them to eat only when they are hungry, which may be quite tricky.

Firstly, they must be able to recognise the signs of hunger, which many Western kids have never experienced. These may include:

- an emptiness in the stomach or 'grumbling'
- lethargy
- tiredness.

They should start feeling hungry after 3 to 4 hours without food. If they have cravings for food in the meantime, suggestions for resisting the urge to eat unnecessarily are on the next page.

Finding distractions

Stress, habit and boredom are the biggest triggers for craving food that the body doesn't need. If your child is pestering for something to eat when she's not actually hungry, then distract her with one or more of the following suggestions (or come up with some of your own, or even ask your child to suggest some) until she is actually hungry and ready to eat, or it's a regular mealtime (whichever comes first):

- Walk the dog
- Call a friend on the cordless phone – and walk while you chat
- Go to the park and kick a ball about
- Practice handstands
- Listen to your favourite music
- Dance
- Have a bath or shower
- Play a board game
- Do a crossword puzzle or Su Doku
- Tidy your bedroom

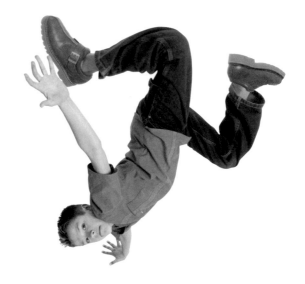

School dinners vs. packed lunches

Schools have made huge strides in their efforts to provide healthier school meals, thanks in large measure to the efforts of Jamie Oliver and other pressure groups. In the vast majority of schools there are usually healthy options on offer now, but whether or not your child is able to discover them in among the tempting faster foods is another question.

There is also a tendency for children to ignore the 'balanced' aspect of choosing their own food. I remember that, on questioning, my younger son told me he had eaten rice and chips for his school dinner because that was all that was left (untrue as it turned out, but it was all that he fancied).

WHEN ENOUGH IS ENOUGH

When your stomach is full, it sends a message to the brain that you are satiated. The problem is that it takes 20 minutes for the message to get through – so, conceivably, you could keep eating for 20 minutes after you're full.

The trick is to get your child to eat slowly – this gives the message time to get through – and to wait before asking for second helpings. After ten minutes or so she may realise that she doesn't actually want anything more.

It may be more work for you but, if you want to keep a greater measure of control over what your child eats, you are best advised to send her to school with a packed lunch. Of course, the biggest challenge to packed lunches, apart from fitting the making of them into an already crammed morning time frame, is to prevent them from becoming monotonous. It's so easy to end up putting the same old things in the box until your bored with it, let alone the kids.

The answer lies in variety and in planning. The first stop is to work out what is needed in the ideal lunch box – and then you can find all manner of exciting items to fill each category.

What goes in the ideal lunch box?

Your child's daily lunch box should contain:

- One carbohydrate food, for example bread, pasta or rice

- One portion of vegetables, for example carrot sticks, cucumber or tomatoes in a sandwich

- One portion of fruit, for example apple, grapes, kiwi fruit cut in half with a spoon or a handful of dried fruit

- One dairy food or calcium-rich food, for example cheese, yoghurt, fromage frais or milk

- One protein-rich food, for example meat, fish, peanut butter, eggs or hummus – usually as a sandwich filling

- A drink, for example ideally a carton of pure fruit juice, water or milk.

Now the exciting bit is to plan a variety of items so that each category is covered and your child's lunch box never becomes dull. You are looking to provide about 200–300 calories in the box each day to give your child enough energy to concentrate through the school lessons.

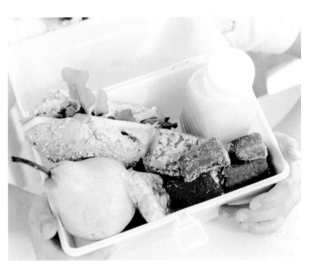

Carbohydrate portion ideas: You could liven up the simple daily sandwich by substituting:

- Pasta, potato or rice salad in a sealed tub
- Tortilla wraps with a favourite filling
- Wholemeal crackers
- Pizza slices
- Mini pittas
- Bagels
- Rolls
- Various types of bread for sandwiches.

Vegetable portion ideas: The vegetable element of a packed lunch can be contained within a sandwich or wrap as part of the filling, or served wrapped separately:

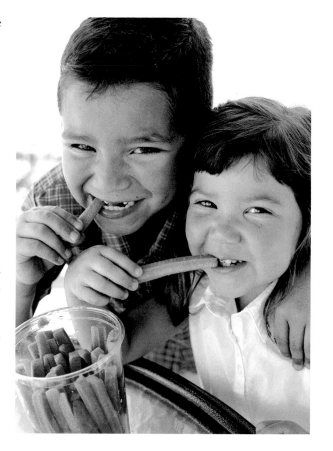

- Tomato, cucumber, lettuce, cress or sweetcorn can be mixed with protein or dairy as a sandwich filling
- Cherry tomatoes
- Cucumber chunks
- Carrot and celery batons
- Red, green, orange and yellow pepper sticks.

Fruit portion ideas: An apple a day might keep the doctor away but it's also pretty dull. Be imaginative with the fruit you include in your child's lunch box and, if she's not a big fan of a piece of fruit per se, you can always slice them up for her or add dried fruit, home-made fruit salads or individual ring-pull tins. Here are some more ideas:

- Apples and pears
- Citrus fruits such as satsumas, clementines or mandarins
- Grapes and cherries (in a pot)
- Kiwi fruit (cut in half and wrapped in cling film, but don't forget the spoon!)
- Peaches and nectarines (these bruise easily so wrap well or, better still, put in a small tub)

■ Dried apricots, mixed fruits, raisins or pineapple.

Dairy portion ideas: These tend primarily to be fillings in sandwiches/wraps etc. but can be stand-alone items too:

■ Cheese (as sandwich filling or in an individual portion)

■ Yoghurt pouches

■ Fromage frais tubes

■ Individual carton of custard.

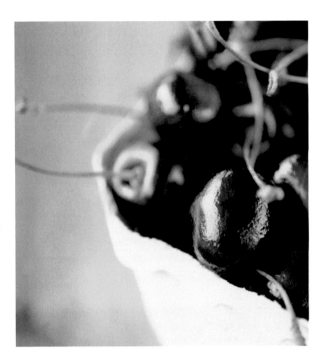

Protein portion ideas: Sandwich fillings and foods include:

■ Cheese

■ Chicken or turkey

■ Ham

■ Tuna

■ Egg

■ Peanut butter

■ A chicken drumstick

■ A cold meat or vegetarian sausage.

Drink ideas: Avoid fizzy drinks and soft drinks but make sure the lunch box has a drink because it's so easy for kids to become dehydrated, which leads to poor concentration, headaches and lethargy. Choose from:

■ Water

■ Milk or milkshake*

■ Fruit juice

■ Probiotic yoghurt drink*

■ Fruit smoothie.*

*With any of these drinks and food items it is important to keep them cool, so an insulated lunch bag or box with a small ice pack is recommended – especially in summer.

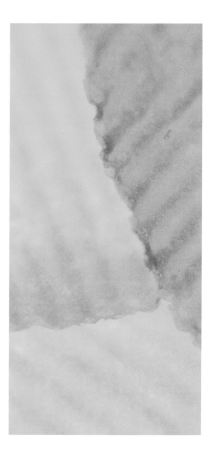

> **tip**
>
> **LUNCH BOX TREATS**
>
> *Occasionally a treat can be added to your child's lunch box as an unexpected surprise – and as long as it's not daily, it won't do any harm. Crisps, cereal bars, chocolate-coated cakes and biscuits are probably the order of the day but, in our household, home-made flapjack, scones or biscuits are just as popular and generally a healthier option.*

Nutrition for older kids

Once your child has moved on to secondary school or into her teens, it is harder for you, as a parent, to control what she eats or to forbid certain foods. While it is still important to promote good habits by eating well yourself and by serving nutritious family meals, your adolescent is able to make her own food choices when she is away from home.

DAILY NUTRITIONAL NEEDS

As teenagers mature, their nutritional requirements become similar to the RDAs for adults. Although teenage girls need fewer calories than teenage boys, an active teen of either gender will need more calories than a sedentary teen. On average, a teenage girl needs 2200 calories per day and a boy, depending on how active he is, needs 2500–3000 calories a day.

Teens need breakfast

When adolescents start self-determining, many try to grab a few extra minutes in bed in the morning by dropping breakfast. However, of the three main daily meals, breakfast is probably the most important for this age group. Teenagers who skip breakfast are:

- less able to concentrate in school
- more likely to eat 'empty' calories during the rest of the day.

Conversely, it has also been shown that youngsters who eat breakfast regularly:

- do better in school
- are more attentive
- eat more healthily generally
- are more likely to be physically active.

If she doesn't want a conventional bowl of cereal (which, by the way, does not have to be limited to breakfast time but makes a great snack for teenagers at any time) then be a bit more innovative in what you have to offer – and let her make it herself!

Here are a few ideas that take no time at all to prepare and may get the ball rolling:

- Fresh fruit smoothies (use semi-skimmed milk, a low fat yoghurt, fresh fruit and crushed ice cubes).
- Open sandwiches with wholemeal bread, meat and cheese.
- Sprinkle grated cheese and sliced tomatoes (or salsa) on a corn tortilla, fold it in half and microwave for 20 seconds.
- Bagels, waffles or crumpets make an interesting alternative to toast – try to liven up the toppings too: why not suggest cream cheese with sliced strawberries?
- Home-made muesli with all her favourite ingredients may tempt her if she's gone off commercial cereals.

Advise rather than dictate

By this age, it is no good dictating to your adolescent what she can and can't eat because it is impossible to police. She is now, inevitably, developing a life independent of you and it is possible that she will rebel against the eating habits instilled by family life. Schools have vending

fact *A study of 4000 British schoolchildren aged 11–12 found that stressed children eat more fatty food, skip breakfast more often and eat fewer fruits and vegetables. The higher the stress levels, the worse the diet becomes.*

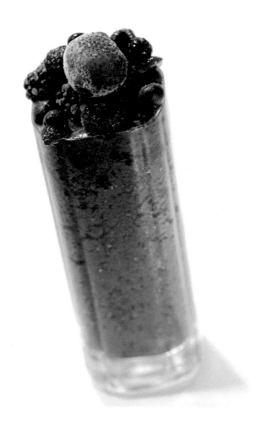

machines full of high-energy snacks and, if the school is wise enough to ban these, there are always shops selling tempting food and drinks on the way to and from school.

The solution is to continue doing what you have done all along and to reinforce the message of healthy eating (without droning on) when appropriate. Statistically, you're on a good bet if you've always practised what you've preached at home, since young kids who eat healthily are known to carry these good eating habits into adulthood. However, here are a few more tricks to help keep your secondary-school kid on the right track:

- Make sure she gets healthy satisfying food at home.
- Encourage her to pack her own (healthy) snacks to get her through the school day.
- Keep the fridge and cupboards stocked with healthy foods and snacks.
- Be aware of your teen's schedule so you can encourage her to have enough sustenance throughout the day and plan meals around her.
- Make family meals a priority.
- Eat well yourself and set a good example.
- Advise her on how to eat sensibly when using school/college canteens.
- Remind her that if she is eating healthy foods for 75–80 per cent of the time (and is active), then she can indulge in a little of what she fancies the rest of the time.

Image-conscious youngsters

In our modern society, the cult of celebrity and the ubiquitous display of perfect airbrushed faces and bodies on advertising pages and hoardings mean that children are more body conscious than ever before, with children as young as eight feeling the need to diet.

They aspire to be thin and beautiful like the film stars and models that they see in magazines, and they believe that they will be happier and more popular if they conform to the right image.

Sadly for these young girls, and increasingly young boys, research shows that those who start dieting before the age of 14 are far more likely to be constantly on diets and to find it hard to maintain a permanent weight. It is believed that early

---

FAST FOOD CHOICES

If your teenager doesn't want to be left out of trips to fast-food restaurants with her mates, then offer these suggestions for how she can minimise the damage:

- Don't go for the super-size or mega-deal options.
- Order fruit juice, water, milk or diet fizzy drinks rather than normal – and get regular rather than large sizes.
- Opt for a grilled chicken sandwich or a veggie-burger.
- Avoid added extras such as cheese, bacon, mayonnaise or sour cream.
- Forget the fries and go instead for baked beans, corn on the cob or salad.

dieting may disrupt the metabolism of teenagers, and the research also shows that, perversely, adolescents who diet are most likely to become obese adults.

This pressure to conform to an artificially thin body image coinciding with new and erratic eating patterns of adolescent and teen years, with the added complication for girls of the onset of puberty (which can mean a change in body shape), may contribute to girls and some boys developing eating disorders in their early teens.

Going to extremes

Between 5 and 10 per cent of adolescent girls show some signs of eating disorders such as anorexia nervosa (severe dieting and weight loss) or bulimia nervosa (bingeing and purging). The incidence of these disorders among boys is negligible.

It is at the stage of puberty when girls are becoming more curvaceous – which many struggle to accept – that these disorders can begin. Young sportswomen who have to be thin for their sport, such as gymnasts and long-distance runners in particular, may dislike the changes to their body shape.

However, severe dieting during puberty can affect growth and delay the onset of menstruation. For those who have already started their periods, these can become erratic or disappear altogether. Both anorexia and bulimia can have serious effects on the long-term health of your child and, in some cases, be life-threatening.

At the first signs of either of these disorders you should seek professional help and advice. Signs of anorexia nervosa include:

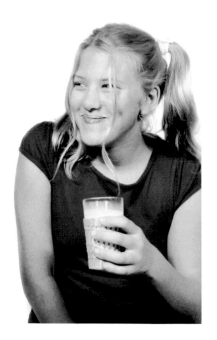

- She expresses dislike of her body image.
- She toys with her food, cuts it into very small pieces and eats very slowly and very little.
- She avoids eating with the family.
- She loses significant weight over a short period of time.
- She wears baggy clothes to cover up and hide her thinness.
- She exercises excessively.
- She is obsessive about calories.
- She weighs herself compulsively – perhaps several times a day – and is distressed by any fluctuation.
- She stops having menstrual periods.

Although much more widespread, bulimia can be harder to spot because there is no drastic weight loss. However, other signs to watch for include:

- Her weight swings up and down by as much as 4.5 kg.

- She spends a lot of time in the bathroom, especially after meals.

- She binge eats without appearing to gain extra weight.

- She complains of sore throats and difficulty swallowing, induced by constant vomiting (tooth enamel can also be damaged).

- She excessively exercises to compensate for overeating.

- She has irregular or absent periods.

FAMILY MEALS

As your adolescent children become more independent, regular shared family meals can be a way of keeping the lines of communication open and an opportunity to make sure that your child is getting the good nutrition that she needs at this crucial developmental stage.

Research carried out in the USA shows that young people, especially adolescent girls, were much less likely to develop eating disorders or to obsess about their weight if they regularly enjoyed eating with their families. They were also more likely to eat fruit and vegetables, rather than snack on high-energy foods, and less likely to become smokers or heavy drinkers.

That news is persuasion enough for most parents, but it's your child that you have to lead to the table, so to speak. Many youngsters are happy eating hunched in front of the television with a plate on their knees or in their rooms listening to music. They will resent being asked to turn off the TV/MP3 player to join the family for dinner, so you will have to make it pretty enticing. Here are a few ideas to get even the most recalcitrant adolescent eating family meals.

- Don't make it into a big deal. It doesn't have to be a three course à la carte affair. A simple supper of salad, bread and cheese will suffice – or even a rare take-away, as long as it's together.

- Invite her friends to dinner occasionally, which may help her to be more enthusiastic.

- Let her choose the menu – she then has a vested interest in sharing the fare.

- Set the table to make it more of a family affair that will appeal to adolescents i.e. candles, flowers, funky cutlery/napkins.

- Get her involved in the preparation, cooking or serving of the meal. Studies show that children are much keener to eat meals they have helped prepare themselves.

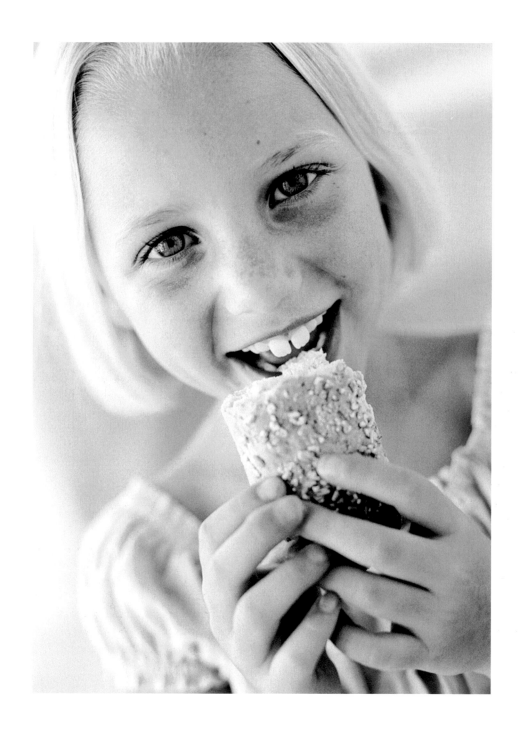

Q&A

Question: I'm worried that my seven-year-old daughter might be taking too much salt. How can I help her to cut down?

Answer: Children who have too much salt can develop health problems such as heart disease and high blood pressure in later life, and they are also more likely to develop a taste for salty foods, which will stay with them when they grow up.
According to the FSA, the maximum amount of salt a child should have depends on their age:

1 to 3 years – 2 g a day (0.8 g sodium)
4 to 6 years – 3 g salt a day (1.2 g sodium)
7 to 10 years – 5 g a day (2 g sodium)
11 and over – 6 g a day (2.5 g sodium)

Babies under a year old should have even less salt.

Around three-quarters of our salt consumption comes from the food we buy, in particular, breakfast cereals, biscuits, soups, sauces, ready-prepared meals, crisps and savoury snacks. So it's important to check labels when shopping. Where possible, choose products that say 'no added salt'.

Another way to reduce the amount of salt your daughter eats is to cut down on salty snacks, such as crisps and salted nuts, and give her low-salt snacks instead. Also curb consumption of burgers, sausages and chicken nuggets, one portion of which contains around half of her daily salt allowance.

Other ways to cut down on salt include:

■ Avoid adding salt to food when you're cooking.

■ Taste food at the table before automatically adding salt.

■ Allow fewer salty foods such as cheese, bacon, pickles and smoked fish.

Question: My thirteen-year-old daughter is a vegetarian. How can I tell if she is eating healthily?

Answer: Teens often voice their independence through the foods they choose to eat and a strong statement is to decide to stop eating meat. However, your daughter can lead a perfectly healthy vegetarian lifestyle but she needs to make sure that she eats a balanced diet. This should be:

■ predominantly starchy foods, such as rice, potatoes, pasta and bread (choosing brown or wholegrain varieties where possible)

■ rich in fruit and veg (at least five portions a day)

■ low in fat and sugar (continued opposite).

Q&A

It's easy for vegetarians to miss out on protein when they give up meat, so make sure your daughter eats plenty of the following each day:

- pulses (such as lentils and beans)
- nuts and seeds
- eggs
- soya products, such as tofu
- milk and dairy products.

Another pitfall for vegetarians, particularly teenage girls, is getting enough iron. This can be found in:

- bread
- fortified breakfast cereals
- green vegetables, such as watercress, broccoli, spring greens and okra
- pulses (namely peas, beans, lentils, peanuts, carob, and soybeans).

It's easier to absorb iron from food when it is eaten with foods containing vitamin C, so it's a good idea to include fruit or vegetables or a glass of fruit juice with an iron-rich meal.

Milk and dairy products are good sources of calcium for vegetarians. Vegans, who don't eat any foods of animal origin, including eggs and milk, should try soya, rice or oats and drinks fortified with calcium instead.

Some vegetarians, especially vegans, don't get enough vitamin B12. Good non-meat and non-dairy sources of this vitamin include yeast extract, fortified bread and fortified breakfast cereals.

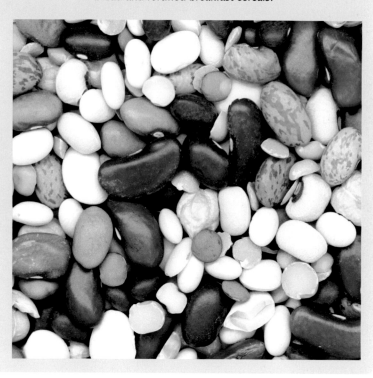

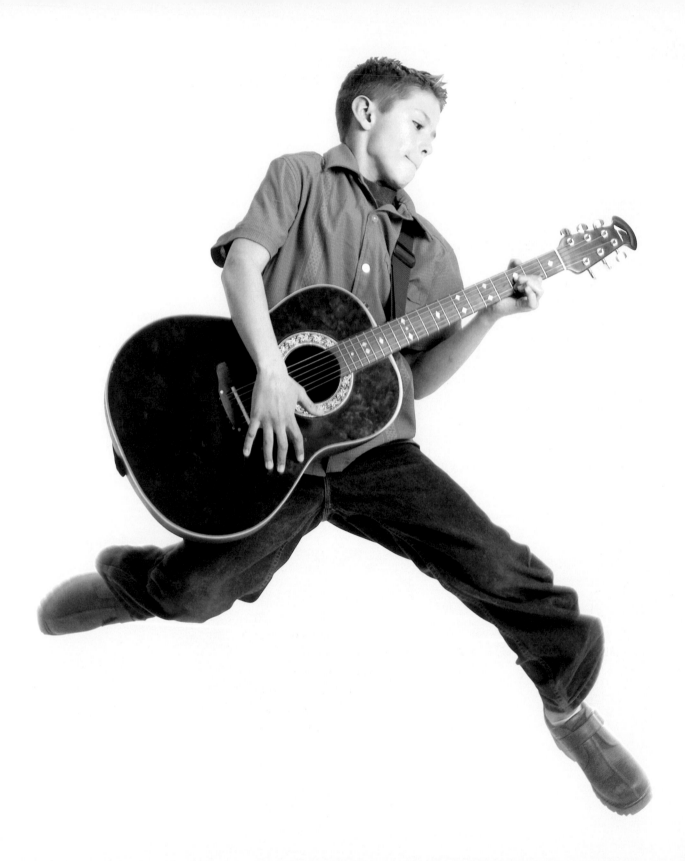

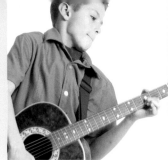

6 activity for big kids

As we have seen from Chapter One, the percentage of overweight children has risen dramatically over the past 30 years. This is worrying not only because of the health problems in adulthood that can ensue from childhood weight problems, but also because of the adverse emotional effect that being overweight can have on our children, which in turn can negatively effect their self-esteem and prospects.

The good news, however, is that overweight kids who want to be more active and achieve a healthy weight have a number of factors working in their favour:

■ Firstly, kids burn a lot of calories just doing the job of growing up, so they have the edge over adults when it comes to weight management.

■ Secondly, we know that the natural inclination of the vast majority of children is to be active – and this is a tendency that you can optimise.

■ Lastly, but definitely not least, they have you! Now, I'd like to spare your blushes but, basically, you cannot underestimate the importance of having interested, supportive parents who want to help. With you on board, offering help and advice on food and activity, and setting an example, your child will stand a far greater chance of becoming more active and of attaining the goal.

The crucial thing is to acknowledge that your child is overweight – and to do so sooner rather than later. It is so much easier to help an infant-school child with a mild weight problem than an obese thirteen-year-old, for example.

In part, this is because pre-teens and younger children are more receptive to parental influence and so it's easier to steer them in the right direction. However, it is also because the social and emotional consequences of being overweight multiply as your child gets older, and so it becomes a bigger problem to handle in an older child.

WHY FAT YOUNGSTERS TURN INTO FAT ADULTS

It is commonly agreed that bad dietary and lifestyle habits formed in childhood are likely to pass with you into adulthood, but there is also a physiological reason why fat youngsters turn into fat adults.

It is during infancy that fat cells are laid down. If fat is stored quickly then additional fat cells are created. As a result, an obese child can have as many as three times the number of fat cells as a normal weight child. Eventually, fat cells lose the ability to multiply and by adulthood you have a fixed number to last you for the rest of your life. The cells you then have simply swell or shrink to accommodate more fat.

Scientists believe that the amount of fat the body stores is proportional to the number of fat cells. So, if you have a higher number to start with (because you were an overweight child) your body is programmed to carry more fat.

Of course, this does not automatically predestine your overweight child to become a fat adult, but he may have to pay more attention as an adult to healthy eating and exercise to maintain a good weight. So, thank goodness he's getting into good habits now.

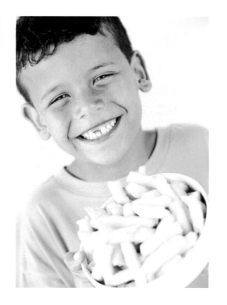

Is my child overweight?

Fooling yourself that your child is just cuddly or big boned, that it's a phase he's going through, or that it's puppy fat and that it will fall off him once he's passed puberty is doing your child no favours at all.

Most parents, if they are honest, know when their child is overweight. However, if you have any uncertainty, the Body Mass Index (BMI) charts (on the following pages) can tell you if there is cause for concern or not.

For most children, BMI is a better indicator than weight alone of whether or not your child is carrying too much body fat because it takes into account height and weight measurements. You can calculate your child's BMI using the following formula:

BMI = (weight in kg ÷ height in cm ÷ height in cm) × 10,000

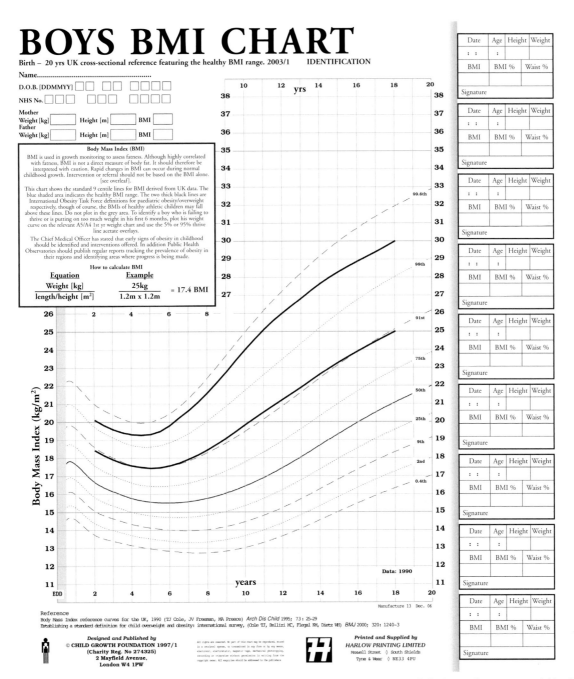

BOYS BMI CHART

Birth – 20 yrs UK cross-sectional reference featuring the healthy BMI range. 2003/1   IDENTIFICATION

Name..

D.O.B. [DDMMYY]

NHS No.

Mother
Weight [kg]   Height [m]   BMI

Father
Weight [kg]   Height [m]   BMI

Body Mass Index (BMI)

BMI is used in growth monitoring to assess fatness. Although highly correlated with fatness, BMI is not a direct measure of body fat. It should therefore be interpreted with caution. Rapid changes in BMI can occur during normal childhood growth. Intervention or referral should not be based on the BMI alone. [see overleaf].

This chart shows the standard 9 centile lines for BMI derived from UK data. The blue shaded area indicates the healthy BMI range. The two thick black lines are International Obesity Task Force definitions for paediatric obesity/overweight respectively, though of course, the BMIs of healthy athletic children may fall above these lines. Do not plot in the grey area. To identify a boy who is failing to thrive or is putting on too much weight in his first 6 months, plot his weight curve on the relevant A5/A4 1st yr weight chart and use the 5% or 95% thrive line acetate overlays.

The Chief Medical Officer has stated that early signs of obesity in childhood should be identified and interventions offered. In addition Public Health Observatories should publish regular reports tracking the prevalence of obesity in their regions and identifying areas where progress is being made.

How to calculate BMI

Equation	Example	
$\dfrac{\text{Weight [kg]}}{\text{length/height [m}^2]}$	$\dfrac{25\text{kg}}{1.2\text{m} \times 1.2\text{m}}$	= 17.4 BMI

Body Mass Index (kg/m²)

years

Data: 1990

Reference
Body Mass Index reference curves for the UK, 1990 (TJ Cole, JV Freeman, MA Preece) *Arch Dis Child* 1995; 73: 25–29
Establishing a standard definition for child overweight and obesity: international survey, (Cole TJ, Bellizzi MC, Flegal KM, Dietz WH) *BMJ* 2000; 320: 1240–3

Manufacture 13 Dec. 06

Designed and Published by
© CHILD GROWTH FOUNDATION 1997/1
(Charity Reg. No 274325)
2 Mayfield Avenue,
London W4 1PW

Printed and Supplied by
HARLOW PRINTING LIMITED
Maxwell Street ◊ South Shields
Tyne & Wear ◊ NE33 4PU

Identification table (repeated blocks):

Date	Age	Height	Weight
: :	:		
BMI	BMI %	Waist %	
Signature			

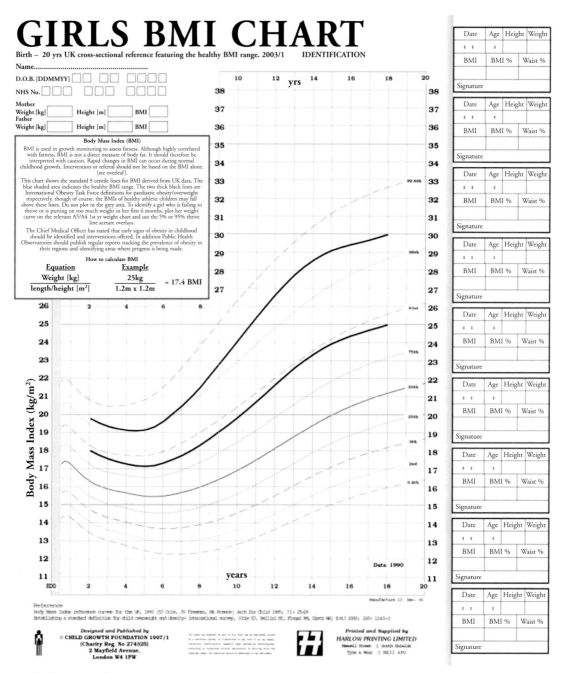

GIRLS BMI CHART

Birth – 20 yrs UK cross-sectional reference featuring the healthy BMI range. 2003/1   IDENTIFICATION

Name..

D.O.B. [DDMMYY]

NHS No.

Mother
Weight [kg]   Height [m]   BMI
Father
Weight [kg]   Height [m]   BMI

Body Mass Index (BMI)

BMI is used in growth monitoring to assess fatness. Although highly correlated with fatness, BMI is not a direct measure of body fat. It should therefore be interpreted with caution. Rapid changes in BMI can occur during normal childhood growth. Intervention or referral should not be based on the BMI alone. [see overleaf].

This chart shows the standard 9 centile lines for BMI derived from UK data. The blue shaded area indicates the healthy BMI range. The two thick black lines are International Obesity Task Force definitions for paediatric obesity/overweight respectively, though of course, the BMIs of healthy athletic children may fall above these lines. Do not plot in the grey area. To identify a girl who is failing to thrive or is putting on too much weight in her first 6 months, plot her weight curve on the relevant A5/A4 1st yr weight chart and use the 5% or 95% thrive line acetate overlays.

The Chief Medical Officer has stated that early signs of obesity in childhood should be identified and interventions offered. In addition Public Health Observatories should publish regular reports tracking the prevalence of obesity in their regions and identifying areas where progress is being made.

How to calculate BMI

Equation	Example	
Weight [kg] / length/height [m²]	25kg / 1.2m x 1.2m	= 17.4 BMI

Body Mass Index (kg/m²)

years

Data: 1990

Reference
Body Mass Index reference curves for the UK, 1990 (TJ Cole, JV Freeman, MA Preece) Arch Dis Child 1995; 73: 25-29
Establishing a standard definition for child overweight and obesity: international survey. (Cole TJ, Bellizzi MC, Flegal KM, Dietz WH) BMJ 2000; 320: 1240-3

Designed and Published by
© CHILD GROWTH FOUNDATION 1997/1
[Charity Reg. No 274325]
2 Mayfield Avenue,
London W4 1PW

Printed and Supplied by
HARLOW PRINTING LIMITED
Maxwell Street () South Shields
Tyne & Wear () NE33 4PU

Date	Age	Height	Weight
BMI	BMI %	Waist %	
Signature			

Date	Age	Height	Weight
BMI	BMI %	Waist %	
Signature			

Date	Age	Height	Weight
BMI	BMI %	Waist %	
Signature			

Date	Age	Height	Weight
BMI	BMI %	Waist %	
Signature			

Date	Age	Height	Weight
BMI	BMI %	Waist %	
Signature			

Date	Age	Height	Weight
BMI	BMI %	Waist %	
Signature			

Date	Age	Height	Weight
BMI	BMI %	Waist %	
Signature			

Date	Age	Height	Weight
BMI	BMI %	Waist %	
Signature			

Date	Age	Height	Weight
BMI	BMI %	Waist %	
Signature			

For example, if your eight-year-old son weighs 27kg and is 128cm tall, then his BMI is:

(27 ÷ 128 ÷ 128) = 0.0016479 × 10,000 = 16.479

Using the BMI chart, you can establish which weight category your son falls into:

- Underweight: less than the 5th percentile
- Ideal weight: between the 5th and 85th percentiles
- At risk of being overweight: between the 85th and 95th percentiles
- Overweight: at the 95th percentile or higher.

For the above example of our hypothetical eight-year-old, you can see that a BMI of 16.5 falls well within the band for ideal weight.

The BMI chart is useful for tracking your child's growth over a period of time and to make sure there are no sudden leaps or troughs. Most children will fall into the 'ideal' BMI category, which is quite broad.

However, don't let the charts lull you into a false sense of security. It is possible that a child can be given an ideal BMI reading but still be at risk of becoming overweight due to poor diet, low activity levels and a family history of weight problems.

Like all charts, BMI should not be followed slavishly but should be used as a helpful guide. However, if your child's reading gives you cause for concern, you can consult your doctor.

Getting the whole family on board

It is almost impossible for your overweight child to go it alone when it comes to changing eating habits and activity levels. It is even more the case than with normal weight kids that it needs to be a whole family approach if he is to succeed.

We have acknowledged that it is not always easy to motivate your child to take on more activity, but if the siblings of an overweight child feel that an increased exercise schedule and healthy diet is being foisted on them simply to support the 'odd one out' then you may be faced with at best resentment, and at worst a refusal to help, or even sabotage.

tip *Try to avoid the knee-jerk reaction to an excess BMI weight reading of putting your youngster straight on a diet (which is not recommended in the majority of cases and certainly not without a nutritionist's guidance). Rather you should use this information as an impetus to kick-start your new approach to healthier living.*

The best approach is to talk openly to the whole family, explaining:

- This is about everyone's health. Steer the focus of attention away from the overweight child.
- That junk food and sweets can damage growth and teeth of thin children as well as those who are overweight.
- Reassure them that the changes are not going to be unpleasant and that doing more together will be fun.
- Offer incentives and rewards to siblings as well as to your overweight child for leading a more active, healthier lifestyle.

United front

Encourage your partner to support your efforts to dump the junk and to do more activities as a family, and make sure you are both agreed that the new healthier living regime is something upon which you will present a united front to the children.

But before you embark on this course, firstly it is worth examining as candidly as possible your own feelings about having an overweight child. Given that we are all conditioned by the media to strive for beauty and lithe bodies, some parents struggle to come to terms with the fact that their child is overweight – especially if they are slim and fit themselves. Some parents confess that they find their overweight child less attractive and feel that he is letting himself and the family down in some way – but that they also feel incredibly guilty for having these thoughts.

In these circumstances, it is worth remembering that disliking your child's current physical appearance is not the same as disliking or not loving your child. Obviously, it is imperative that your child does not get wind of your distaste at all. And it is also important that you use these negative emotions to spur you on to help him to be more active.

fact *According to government research, one-third of Scottish twelve-year-olds are overweight and one-fifth are obese, compared to one-sixth in the USA and one in twenty across Britain as a whole – making Scottish kids the fattest children in the world.*

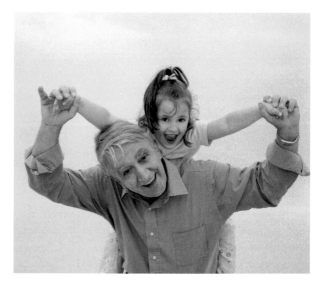

Peter Mackreth, Senior Lecturer in Physical Activity and Obesity Management at Leeds Metropolitan University, finds it is more common for parents of overweight kids to feel guilty and to blame themselves for their child's situation. He says, 'Very often, the parents are overweight or obese themselves. They are guilty and slightly shameful. But who's really to blame if parents are not educated to know what to do.' (For more details, see page 121 for information on weight loss camps).

Giving the right signals

Wherever you find yourself on this emotional spectrum, there are a few ways in which you can feel more comfortable about your response to your child's body weight, and adapt your attitude to best help your child:

- **Remember his basic shape is genetic**: Your child can become more toned, fitter and lead a healthier lifestyle but he cannot change his basic body type. If you dreamed of having a long, lean athletic son when he is short-limbed and stocky, just like all the Smiths before him, then you are in for a disappointment. Get over it – it's not his fault.

- **Being overweight does not make your child a bad or unattractive person**: Let your child know that you love him for who he is, no matter what his size or shape.

- **Focus on the good points**: If you struggle emotionally with having an overweight child, then distract yourself from his weight by focussing on his strengths and praising them, and by positively helping him to become more active and to eat more healthily.

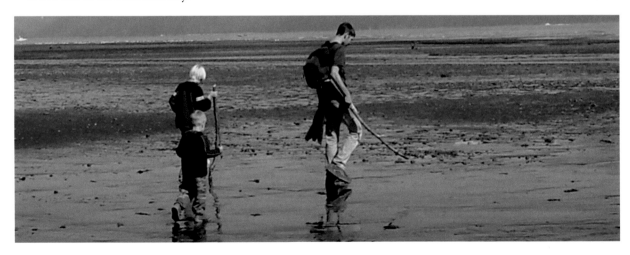

■ **Hide your disappointment**: Otherwise, if your son senses that you blame him for his weight because you feel perhaps that he has no willpower, is lazy or is greedy, then he may well compensate for what he probably sees as disapproval or a withdrawal of your affection by comfort eating – a common response in unhappy children.

■ **Dump the guilt**: Beating yourself up because your child is overweight or blaming him is counter productive. Instead, start looking for positive solutions.

■ **Be patient**: For change to be adopted permanently it is best introduced gradually. Don't be extreme in introducing new regimes.

■ **Change your priorities**: The emphasis is on eating healthy food and building more activity into your lives – not on weight.

■ **Be kind to yourself**: When progress appears agonisingly slow, remind yourself that you are doing things the best way possible for the emotional and physical well-being of your child.

Activities for big kids

It can be a vicious circle for overweight kids. They feel self-conscious about exercising (perhaps they do not want to change in front of the other kids, or feel conspicuous in swimming trunks) and they may also feel that they are doomed to make a fool of themselves or to fail. So they retreat and do less and less activity, which in turn adds to their weight problems.

As Peter Mackreth points out,

'In this country we're very good at providing new opportunities for children already engaged in physical activities but not very good at providing opportunities for those who are inactive. We need to offer things for children who don't want to be involved in competitive sport.'

You can be sensitive to these exercise concerns, but don't cave in. You have to reassure your child and stress the amazing benefits that he will reap from being active. And then find positive ways to help him to get started.

fact *According to the British Nutrition Foundation, the diets of British 4-year-olds in the 1990s contained less iron, less energy and more sugar than in 1950s Britain.*

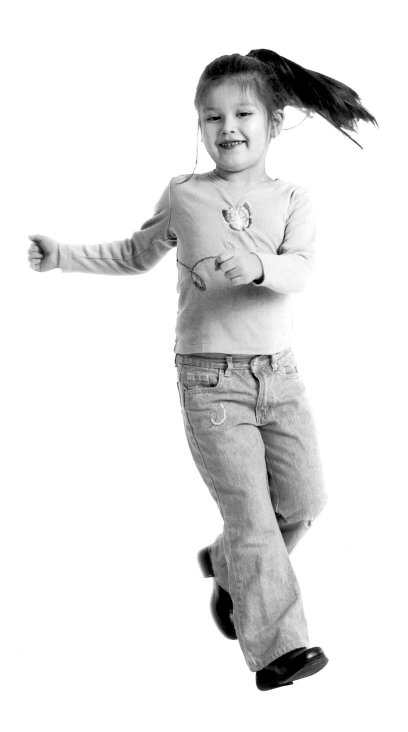

FIT VS. FAT

Unless your child is extremely overweight or obese, in which case specialist nutritional help is available, you should not put your child on a diet. Dramatically cutting calorie intake or cutting out certain food groups can be damaging to your child's health and it could impede his growth or natural development.

Diets also cause:

- tiredness

- fatigue

- poor concentration in school – they need enough fuel to be able to concentrate all day.

It is more important to teach your child the value of healthy eating and being active. Then your child will naturally end up in the right weight range using gradual lifestyle changes rather than dieting to hit a target weight.

A combination of improved eating habits and increased activity will be enough to give your child moderate weight loss, or to maintain his weight so that, as he grows taller, he appears slimmer and trimmer.

The scientific reasons why physical activity should be part of any weight management initiative are:

- Activity helps preserve muscle mass. If your child goes on a reduction diet without activity, he will lose muscle mass (you burn protein from muscle in response to a drastic reduction in calories) as well as fat.

- He is more likely to maintain weight loss if physical activity is included in his weight loss intervention.

- As your child increases his fitness level, so he has a better chance of continuing to lose weight because he has a greater muscle mass and therefore activity becomes easier and, ipso facto, he is more likely to enjoy it.

- Also, greater lean body mass increases the metabolism, so the more muscle he has, the more calories he'll burn just sitting around.

- Exercise helps his body burn extra calories even after he's finished because the increase in his base metabolic rate (BMR) due to activity can last from 6 to 24 hours after 30 minutes of moderate exercise.

- It is possible to be overweight and fit and have a lower mortality rate than someone who is of normal weight and unfit. Therefore, if you do physical activity you will increase your fitness levels and improve your health.

Here are some ideas:

- Research shows that individual goal-based sports can be better for overweight children than competitive team sports, particularly when they are getting started. So suggest individual activities that may interest him – swimming, archery, golf, tennis, martial arts, ice skating etc. – and get him to set personal goals such as quicker length times or a lower golf round.

- Walking and swimming are good for overweight kids because they are kinder to the joints. High-impact activities can be difficult.

- If he fancies a team sport, choose one that plays to his strengths i.e. favours strength over speed. Korfball is a great choice for those who don't like rough team sports (see box on page 120).

- Sometimes private tuition or small private classes can be a great boost to help your child catch up on a skill and develop enough confidence to join a large group class or team.

- If he is self-conscious about his appearance, let him choose and buy the appropriate sports clothing and trainers that he will feel good about wearing. Make sure it gives adequate support and don't fob him off with an old baggy T-shirt that covers his size but ends up making him stand out from his peers.

- Make realistic goals. What seems like small potatoes to you may be a challenge to an overweight child (you'd be surprised how much effort is involved in the smallest movements when you are carrying extra weight). Set modest challenges, for example increasing the time he is able to walk briskly by a minute a day until he reaches his daily target of 30 minutes.

- Until your child is comfortable exercising or playing sport in public, why not get some home equipment such as a mini-bouncer or rowing machine, so he can start to get fit at home. Similarly, an age-appropriate exercise video might prove popular.

- Your overweight child is at greater risk of dehydration when he exerts himself, so make sure he has plenty of water on hand.

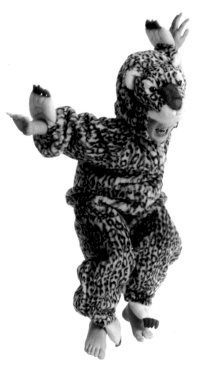

- He is also more prone to injury, so emphasise the need for warm-up and cool-down sessions before sport or strenuous activity.

- He will respond well if you praise his efforts to get active, however modest they may appear.

Remember, the key is not 'do as I say', but 'do as I do'. So get out there with him, and play together. You know the deal by now – whatever you find fun: frisbee, badminton, a walk along the cliffs, feeding the ducks at the park. He's burning calories doing all these activities and any more that you care to come up with. Remember, your child doesn't have to work himself into a lather for activity to be beneficial.

tip *Whatever your child's size, individual pursuits such as swimming or cycling have the advantage that they can continue as a lifelong passion well into adulthood. Sadly, most team sports fall by the wayside once we become adults so it is good to encourage a combination of team and individual sports in your child's repertoire.*

KORFBALL

This is the fastest-growing sport in Europe and is a cross between netball and basketball. The teams are mixed gender and it is tactical. Everyone gets a chance to defend and attack because team members swap positions and, since you are not allowed to run with the ball, there's no physical contact. Another attraction for the overweight player is that most games last around 15 minutes only. So, they can keep going without losing performance and can build stamina in the process.

WEIGHT LOSS CAMPS

The international Carnegie Weight Loss Camps, developed at Leeds Metropolitan University, are the only scientifically proven weight loss camps for overweight young people in the world.

The physical activity and healthy eating programmes promote an immediate and safe weight loss during the camp. In addition, a child-centred approach provides positive experiences of physical activity, lifestyle education and social interaction promoting lifestyle changes for long-lasting results at home.

Co-founder, Pete Mackreth, explains:

"What we deliver is good quality inclusive, age- and developmentally-appropriate activity. We ensure all kids involved have "opportunities to be successful".

Then they feel they should be there. If they are more confident, they are more likely to have fun and engage with it, and so are more likely to continue. We have never worked with any child who has not been able to do physical activity – and last year, our biggest teenage boy weighed 42 stone.'

The residential summer camp is for 11 to 17-year-olds and there are 150 places. Children have to be overweight to attend. It costs £3000 for 8 weeks (which is a subsidised price. According to Mackreth, you'd pay at least £2000 more for a similar camp in the USA).

As well as the camps, Carnegie Weight Management runs community treatment programmes, awareness campaigns and education and training programmes. (For contact details, see Useful contacts on pages 145–50).

If you are considering what's euphemistically known as a 'fat camp' for your child, you must assure yourself of one or two points before coming to a decision:

- Both you and your child must view the camp in a wholly positive light. If your child needs to be coerced or views attendance as some kind of punishment, a camp should not be considered.

- Is your child committed to making changes in his lifestyle?

- Are you confident that he is mature enough to be away from home for a number of weeks?

- Can you afford to pay out this amount of money when there is no iron-cast guarantee of success?

- Are you emotionally prepared if it does not work long term? Will you blame your child?

- Are you happy to hand over responsibility for your child's weight loss to someone else without feeling that you have failed in some way or feeling guilty?

Emotional fallout

Without doubt, there are physical disadvantages that overweight children have to overcome. However, for many young people, the greatest burden of being overweight is the emotional and social damage that often ensues.

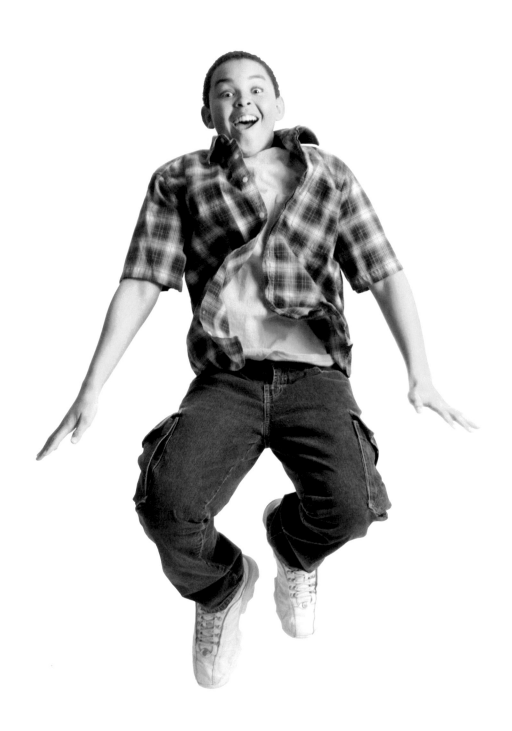

In today's society, where physical perfection and beauty are so highly prized, the overweight child can be ridiculed and abused by his peers. Typically, as a result, his confidence will be low (or certainly knocked), and many overweight children become worried, self-critical and depressed.

Overweight children of all ages can be the victims of teasing but it can often be at its worst during adolescence. The social difficulties caused by being overweight can drive some kids to even greater problems. It is no coincidence that overweight children are more prone to depression and risky behaviours such as self-harming, drug and alcohol abuse.

Nonetheless, you are already taking the most important step in helping your overweight child by setting him on a path to a healthier lifestyle. However, in the interim, there are also ways in which you can help him to deal with the emotional fallout of being overweight, until he reaches his goal of a healthier, fitter body:

Acknowledge your child's weight problem: Accepting that he has a weight problem is your child's first step to overcoming the situation. If he is in denial, he is unable to make changes or to deal effectively with the teasing, and its emotional repercussions.

Build self-esteem: Although you cannot bear full responsibility for your child's self-esteem, what you say and your attitudes to weight and exercise have a huge bearing on how your child feels about himself.

For instance, discussing his weight issues in front of other people, nagging him about how much he's eating, giving him a smaller slice of birthday cake than his siblings, or pitying his sports performance are all ways in which inadvertently you could be damaging your child's self-esteem.

You can try to bolster low self-esteem or maintain your child's good self-image by:

- Recognising his strengths and talents and praising them.
- Being sincere. You don't have to tell him he's great at something he's not. Children can smell insincerity a mile off. Be honest but avoid negative or derogatory comments. If he asks you straight out, 'Am I fat?' you need to be able to answer positively, along the lines of: 'You are carrying a little extra weight. It's no big deal though because you're doing something about it, and I'm going to help you.'

- Conveying your values to your child. Occasional comments such as, 'You look nice in that', or 'That was a good joke. You've got a good sense of humour', is enough to build confidence in their appearance and abilities and assures them that you value qualities other than just beauty or sporting prowess.

- Reassuring him. It is ok to acknowledge that your child is overweight as long as you make it clear that this is purely a matter of a difference in appearance, just as some children are tall and some are short. It has no bearing whatsoever on a person's character or value.

Talk to other family members: Criticisms and insensitive remarks from members of the family can be extremely damaging. Make it clear to siblings that hurtful or snide comments about weight will not be tolerated.

Similarly, extended members of the family need to know that the issue is in hand and what approach you are taking. Grandparents are notorious for putting their foot in it – so have a quiet word with them and explain that telling your son that 'he'll never get a girlfriend if he doesn't lose some weight' is not helpful.

Talk about society's views: Although you cannot change society's response to overweight people, you can reinforce certain messages that will help your child to maintain good self-esteem in the face of other kids' negative comments.

- Explain that the images you see in magazines and films are unrealistic and unhealthy. In fact, research proves that only 1 in 10,000 women are physically able to attain the stick-thin body of a model.

- Stress that beauty has more to do with qualities such as kindness, being helpful and fairness than good looks and being thin. 'Beauty is only skin deep' is a good adage to reinforce these values.

- Reiterate that you don't have to be thin to get the things you want in life.

- And most important of all, you cannot point out too many times that it is more important to eat healthily and be active than to look like a model.

Make the distinction between being popular and friendship: We have seen that kids often discriminate against overweight children. Being shunned or teased by the 'popular' kids means that overweight children do not feel accepted or that they fit in. During school, being accepted by your peers and being popular are hugely important. So, while acknowledging the pressure that he faces, it is key that your child understands that enjoying good friendships (however few) is more rewarding than being popular – and that he can be happy and successful and have good friends without ever being popular.

If your child is gauche and finds it hard to make friends, you can help him to improve his social skills by:

- Welcoming his friends into your home.
- Supporting his social activities by offering lifts.
- Inviting his friends to come along when you take part in family activities.
- Encouraging him to join a team or take part in a class. It's an opportunity to meet other kids, and being part of a team while having fun can improve confidence in social situations.

Give him coping strategies: If your child is being teased or bullied because of his size, then he needs some strategies to deal with the taunts.

- Explain that reacting to bullies by crying or becoming upset only encourages them. He should try not to react to the bullies' taunts. If bullies can't goad the victim into a response, they'll get bored.
- Practise assertiveness techniques – see websites in Useful contacts (pages 145–50) for details.
- Help your child think up simple responses to the bullies' taunts. It doesn't have to be brilliantly witty but victims report that it helps to have a reply prepared.
- Tell him to find a close friend who will support him and make him feel better and to keep as far away as possible from known tormentors.
- Try to minimise opportunities for bullying i.e. help him to buy clothes that make him look his best in terms of style and colour, give tips on getting changed into PE kit without revealing too much etc.

tip **DON'T WORRY, BE HAPPY**

Research shows that optimism and perseverance are key qualities in the lives of successful people. Whether your child was born believing the cup was half-empty or half-full, these are qualities that he can acquire, and ones that will stand an overweight child in good stead in facing life's challenges.

You can promote his optimism and resilience by:

- *encouraging him to be the best he can be, not necessarily the best.*
- *surrounding him with adults who believe in him and want the best for him.*
- *keeping him active and interested.*
- *being upbeat yourself and demonstrating an 'I'll give it a go' mentality.*
- *showing that you stick at things, even if you find it hard going.*
- *having fun as a family.*

fact *Research suggests that there is a connection between loneliness, boredom and over-eating. Home alone kids who raid the fridge in the hours between getting home from school and parents returning from work are probably doing so because they are on their own and feeling lonely and/or bored. If your child falls into this category, an after-school programme has been proven to prevent this cycle.*

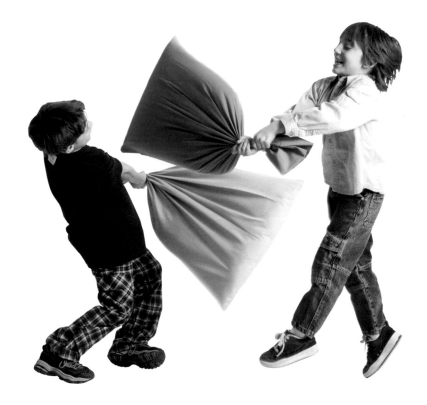

Dealing with depression

Research shows that only 3–6 per cent of 14–16 year olds suffer from true depressive illness and depression is rare in children under the age of 9. However, if your child is consistently miserable, withdrawn and depressed and it lasts for more than 2 or 3 weeks, then you may have cause for concern.

tip *Overweight children often rush through their meals. You can help him to put the brakes on by getting your child to eat with his non-dominant hand. Swapping his knife and fork to the other hand automatically slows the rate at which your child eats. Similarly, chewing each mouthful 15–30 times or putting down cutlery between each bite are tricks that also work.*

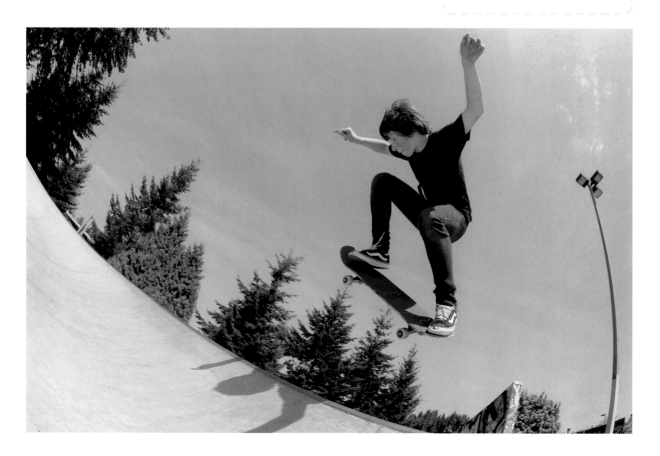

How to spot a depressed teenager

According to the charity YoungMinds, it is important to know the difference between teenage blues and serious depression. If your overweight youngster has experienced three or more of these symptoms and has felt like it for more than two weeks, go and see your doctor or contact one of the organisations listed in Useful contacts (pages 145–50):

- complains of boredom
- low energy and feeling tired all the time
- nothing feels good any more
- lack of interest in food or overeating
- loss of interest in school or friends
- irritability, agitation and uncharacteristic outbursts of anger or aggression
- great anxiety
- no interest in normal social/sporting activities
- decrease in self care
- sleeping too much or too little
- requesting frequent days off school
- difficulty concentrating
- feeling guilty about things
- feeling life is pointless
- lack of sex drive
- tearfulness.

Much as you want to help your child yourself, if he is truly under the influence of depression, you can't do it alone. He needs to seek professional help – preferably your family doctor who may prescribe anti-depressants, but the first-line treatment for youngsters (as long as the waiting list isn't too long) is usually some kind of psychological treatment – either counselling or psychotherapy.

fact *Did you know that comfort eating has a scientific explanation? Stress causes serotonin levels in the blood to drop, which causes cravings for carbohydrates. Those who are sad or stressed turn to carb-laden foods such as sweets for instant comfort, but this perpetuates the problem, as the comfort eating piles on the pounds, and so it goes on.*

Q&A

Question: My 13-year-old daughter is being teased at school because she is overweight. She has started to starve herself to lose weight, but I'm concerned that there may be side effects from such sudden weight loss in a girl her age. Should I be worried?

Answer: Extreme calorie reduction is never a good idea, and dieting is not recommended for children. Your daughter will be losing fat but she will also be losing muscle and potentially damaging her growth. She is likely to become lethargic and bad tempered. She could also become light-headed and dehydrated.

Question: We are keen to introduce our overweight son to sport. Are there any sports that he should avoid?

Answer: Be guided by your son and ask what he is drawn to. There are no sports that are out of bounds to an overweight child. However, as a broad generalisation, overweight kids find running hard, so when choosing a sport perhaps you should avoid sports that involve a lot of running e.g. football, hockey or basketball.

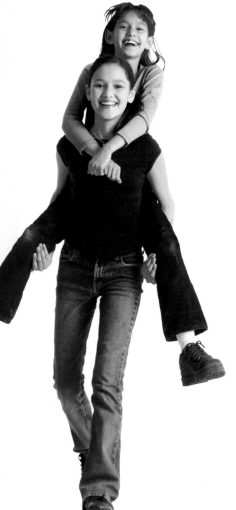

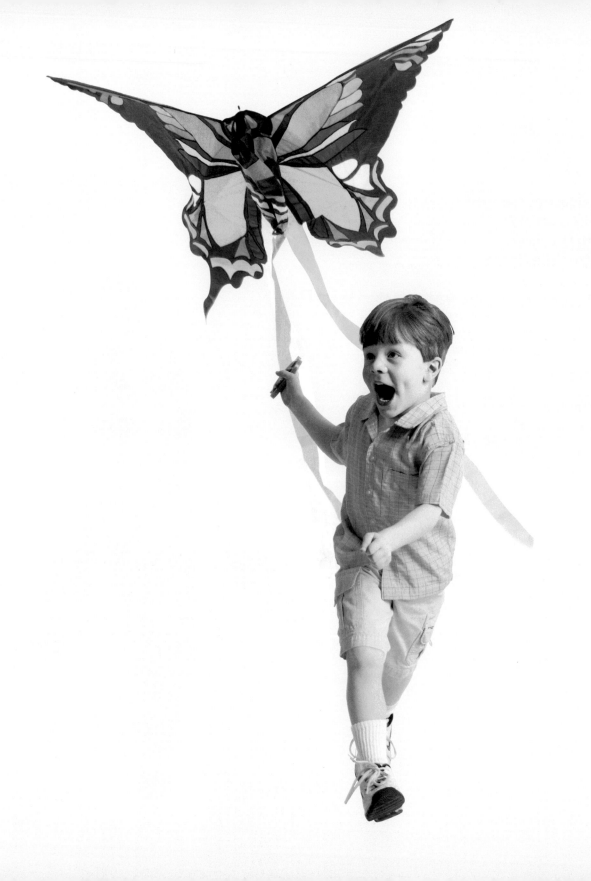

7 staying the course

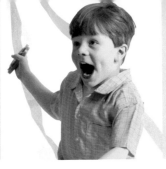

Once you have felt the benefits of a more active lifestyle, then it is hard to give them up and revert to your previously sedentary ways.

However, it would be naive to think that there are not enormous pressures and temptations in modern living that can jeopardise your good intentions. During stressful and pressurised periods it is easy for family activities, or your own personal fitness regime, to slip down the list of priorities.

As your children become older and more independent, so it becomes harder to juggle their commitments and social life with your own – and still fit in time to do things together.

The only effective answer is to be aware of the dangers and to be vigilant. Stand firm against the pressure to submit to outside forces such as children's peer pressure to be 'cool', ergo 'inactive', the lure of convenience foods, or the attraction of quick fixes – the list is endless and relentless.

It is possible to stick with your new-found healthier and more active lifestyle – and because they have started younger, your children stand a greater chance of adopting these attitudes as an accepted part of their lives – forever.

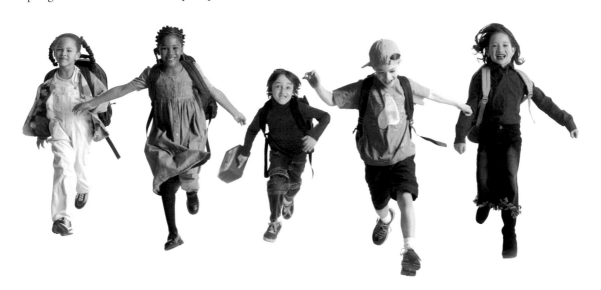

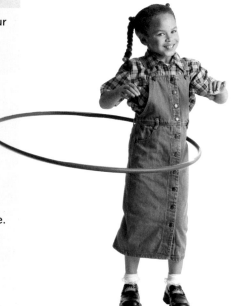

KEEPING IT UP

Make a supreme effort to resist outside pressures that prevent you and your family from leading an active lifestyle. Keep these few suggestions as golden rules to bolster your resolve:

- Eat together as a family whenever possible, and at least twice a week.

- Prioritise exercise and build extra time into your daily schedule for walking rather than driving.

- Keep one weekly session of family activity together as sacrosanct – perhaps a Sunday afternoon.

- If your kids' friends hold sway over them, then invite their friends to join you in your family activity – say a joint game of tenpin bowling, for example.

- Look at family holidays and breaks that involve activity rather than lying by a pool, for example water sports, skiing, walking, hiking, cycling etc.

- Remind yourself that you're doing the best for your family, while still having fun.

Long-lasting changes

Until healthy living is second nature to you and your family (and none of us can rest on our laurels) you have to stay focused on your role as chief whip in the house. It will fall to you to chivvy dissenters and those who are slipping back into their old ways. You are the one who has to continue to rally the troops for family activities and fun outings. And it's you who has the primary role of providing healthy meals and snacks to fuel everyone's new healthy living regime.

So, if you're finding the role of advocate and example-setter is beginning to wear thin, here are the famous five top tips to keep you upbeat and on track:

1. **Focus on the positives**: It's human nature to notice the failings and faults in your loved-ones, and to react to them. But it is less common for us to comment or praise the small but important steps that our children make towards positive lifestyle changes. So save your energy.

Try to ignore or play down slips in the new healthy living routine (one blow-out day fuelled with fizzy drinks and sweets won't do any harm in the great scheme of things) and instead reward your child with positive attention, praise and small treats for doing something right (don't exclude yourself in this reward scheme – all adults appreciate a little self-reward too, you know).

Noticing the fact that your son elected to join you for a walk with the dog rather than watching TV is the best way to keep everyone positive about living more healthily. Remember, your key role is to be positive and upbeat, encouraging and empathetic. It is to bolster your family's resolve and to help your child to believe that the changes he is making are worthwhile. So:

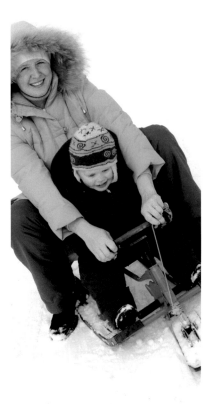

- bite back the criticism if he occasionally slips up (as he undoubtedly will)
- help him to identify healthier options
- acknowledge his success when he gets it right.

2. **Team effort**: Although you are the main protagonist in instigating these changes, don't lose sight of the fact that you have all signed up to the new house rules on healthy eating and being more active.

It may well be you who spots the slide in everyone's good intentions, but it is not up to you to solve the problem alone. You point out the trend and then find solutions as a family.

3. **Quality time**: Hateful phrase, I know – and the bane of most parents' lives. Nevertheless, I cite it here because you need to put the emphasis on quality.

We all know it's hard to fit everything in and that, sometimes, other commitments/tasks may have to fall by the wayside in order to spend more time being active and having fun as a family. But if you resent every moment that you spend playing tennis with your child or cycling with the family, for example, because you could be doing something else, then it is not quality time and it will not be fun for anyone. And then it becomes harder to maintain the momentum of your new initiative.

If you've put all this effort into carving out time for you and the family, you should at least make the most of it and have some fun. Time invested in your child now – *without* the tell-tale whiff of burning martyr or 'look at the sacrifices I'm making for you' sour look on your face – will forge stronger family bonds and have a positive impact on areas of your family life that you could not necessarily have foreseen at the start.

4. Keep some perspective: Sometimes you have to remind yourself that small steps in the right direction are the best way forward for sustainable change. Your child doesn't have to be running marathons or eating the perfect diet. He only has to take enough small steps on the road to healthier living to achieve his goal.

5. Be kind to yourself: It is proven that parents are better able to affect change in their children's life than in their own. And that's because we care about our children's future and put our own needs lower down the list of priorities.

Of course it is only right and natural that you invest in your child but you must also care for yourself. You are making healthier choices to benefit your child's future but don't forget that you will also feel better for the changes. And since we have seen how important being a role model is for our children, do not neglect your own health and fitness requirements.

Progress check

Whether your new more active lifestyle is working well, or whether your family is sliding into old sedentary ways, it can be worth checking every so often to evaluate progress.

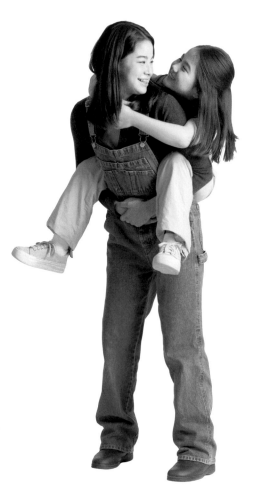

- An informal family discussion in which you praise the efforts and acknowledge the good work of family members will help to keep the positive momentum going.

- Give your child an opportunity to have his say. This is particularly important for adolescents and teenagers who are seeking autonomy. Expressing what is working for them and why and, conversely, what is not, helps them to feel they have some control over the changes in their life.

- Remain calm if your child harps on about what he misses from his previous lifestyle. It's natural for him to vent a little – it doesn't actually mean that he is going to revert to old ways.

- If things are not going as well as you hoped, try and establish why. Is there too much change too quickly? Are there enough low-fat, low-calorie snacks available to replace the banned high-fat, high-calorie items?

- Once you've identified areas of difficulty, ask for potential solutions and present some of your own.

- Ask what more can be done to support the new healthy initiative and if there are any more things that the family would like to do in the way of activity. Perhaps there's a day out they'd love to experience or an activity they'd like to try that you hadn't thought about.

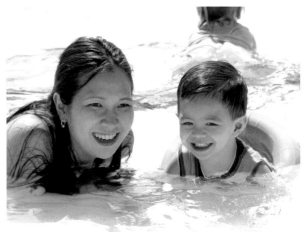

- Conclude by raving about the things you've enjoyed since you've all been more active. Perhaps you love your higher energy levels. Or maybe you feel trimmer and firmer as a result of more activity and a healthier diet. Your positive approach can greatly influence your child's perception, so don't hesitate to:

  - recap on how much you've all achieved so far

  - remind everyone of all the reasons for wanting to change in the first place

  - reiterate your support for everyone and tell them how much you appreciate their continued support and encouragement.

Look how far you've come

It's easy to forget how much progress you have made as a family when you are making gradual lifestyle changes. After all, well-being and good general health are hard to evaluate.

On reflection, your child might be able to comment that he has more energy or you might notice that your skin and hair look healthier, or maybe your partner's clothes hang better than before. Yet, these benefits are not so conspicuous that people would stop any of you in the street and remark on them.

Perhaps for the sake of younger members of the family, who like things to be quantifiable, it is worth finding a way of measuring the benefits of your more active way of life. Why not find an area of fitness that features in your

tip *Pick a relaxed time to hold a progress meeting. If you pick a pressurised time – for example, you've just had a falling-out or your son's favourite TV show is about to be screened – then the meeting will be doomed to failure or, at best, you'll get some sullen, inaccurate and unrepresentative feedback.*

child's new lifestyle and measure his progress in that particular field. Perhaps, at the outset, your child could only swim two lengths of the local pool. Some weeks in to the new regime he might well be able to double that number. If he's playing a sport that is improving his general fitness levels, you can demonstrate this to him by timing how long it takes him to run the length of the local playing field at regular intervals – say once a month – and see his time improve. If running is not his bag, then count the number of sit-ups he can do month by month.

These demonstrable signs of improvement are highly motivating, whatever your age, and easier to understand than vague notions of 'feeling better for it'.

Enlisting support

If the novelty of greater activity starts to wear off, shore up family resolution by getting others on board:

■ Ask friends and relatives to join you in some of your family activities.

■ Involve people that your child likes and respects and with whom he would like to spend more time – and remember that your presence is not always essential. Perhaps he could play a round of golf with a favourite uncle – it can be much more of a temptation or treat to do an activity with a well-liked adult rather than his well-loved but familiar parents.

■ One of my sons still talks about the occasion when a friend's father took him fishing for the first time one day. He caught an eel and was delighted – but what made it so special was that he had been singled out to spend time with a well-liked adult on his own.

■ Make sure that family, friends and exercise professionals are aware of your child's increased efforts to be active and that they offer praise and support whenever possible.

■ Elderly relatives may no longer be fit enough to be involved physically by kicking a ball around the garden, or some other equivalent, but they can play an important role in boosting confidence and self-esteem and encouraging greater participation in sports and outdoor activities by showing an interest.

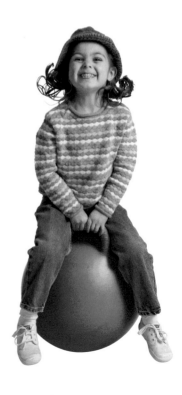

PARENTAL BURNOUT

For all parents, and especially for single parents, assuming the responsibility for your family's fitness and good health can be time-consuming and relentless. If you are spreading yourself thinly between work, social and domestic commitments, and also devoting more time to being active with your kids, then you can expect to feel stretched.

Sometimes, however, parents take on too much and end up feeling burnt-out. You can guard against this by taking these few simple precautions:

- Surround yourself with a support network of friends, family, coaches, instructors and teachers who can shoulder some of the responsibilities.

- Make life easier for yourself by befriending other parents involved in the same activities as your child and sharing lifts etc.

- Enlist the help of local initiatives, clubs and community facilities to provide opportunities for fun and fitness for your child.

- Encourage your child to seek out other active kids who want to participate in activities or come and play in your garden/local park, depending on age.

tip EXPERT'S TIP

Peter Mackreth, Senior Lecturer in Physical Activity and Obesity Management at Leeds Metropolitan University, suggests that your child is more likely to stick at an activity if he feels competent. So choose an activity that he will want to continue. He says,

'Don't just do an activity because it is good for you because you're more likely to give up on that. Find something that you enjoy and want to do and you will feel empowered to continue.'

Falling off the wagon

There will inevitably be periods in your family life when you are not able to honour all of your new healthier lifestyle commitments. There are bound to be occasional slip-ups in diet or activity plans. But, rather like riding a horse, when you fall off you have to get straight back in the saddle, so to speak.

So, if you have an unexpected weekend of slobbing out in front of your favourite DVDs and forego your normal Sunday trip to the park, that's ok. Don't feel too guilty – but make sure you go the next week.

The danger lies in a gradual and unremarked decline back into a sedentary lifestyle. To continue the analogy, if

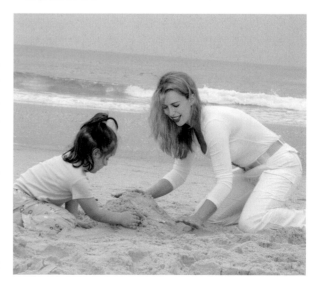

you miss the Sunday outing several weeks on the trot it is easy to believe that it's not worth the hassle of getting back into the habit again.

So, be vigilant against a gradual slide and, where possible, be proactive and positive about rest periods.

Taking a break

If you know that you or your child have a hectic few days/weeks ahead of you, then consciously say that you will miss your trips to the pool this week. After all, you do not want your exercise commitments to become yet one more pressure that you feel you have to honour and that simply adds to your stress levels.

Rather, you can make clear to everyone how much you have missed your weekly swim and how much you're looking forward to getting back to it once the end of year accounts are finished at the end of this month, or when Aunty Hilda's visit is over or whatever the source of your particularly busy period might be.

Similarly, if your child has a week of evening performances at the school concert coming up, don't beat yourself up (or him, figuratively speaking) for missing his sports club that week and for shelving the family outing. This holds true for all periods of busy or stressful pressure in his life. But it is worth noting that if you're thinking about abandoning physical activity commitments at exam time, that exercise is one of the best releases for stress, and that a game of football might be just the break from revision that he needs.

And, in the meantime, although you may have temporarily shelved your major activity plans, you don't have to abandon the everyday ways in which you were building more activity into your lives such as taking the stairs rather than the lift etc. – remember?

Outside pressures

Our youngsters are bombarded with thousands of conflicting messages and facts about the latest diet, health and fitness news – some of it of merit, most of it not. Magazines, books, TV, the Internet, teachers and peers – they will hear advice from every quarter, and many of the messages are very seductive. What star-struck adolescent would not be tempted by a 'guaranteed' quick-fix diet and exercise video from their latest celebrity idol?

ACTIVITY DIARY

Some people who have made long-term lifestyle changes for their family recommend keeping an 'activity diary' to help keep your ambitions on track. Initially, supporters recommend doing a seven-day diary and then cutting down to three days a week, but many fans confess that, just like Bridget Jones, an activity diary becomes compulsive and an integral part of their day.

So, on a daily basis, note all your activities, including day-to-day things such as 25 minutes walking to work or 15 minutes spent ironing, as well as the more structured activities such as 40 minutes swimming.

Older children can also benefit from keeping a diary – it helps not only in monitoring progress but also in identifying what might be happening to prevent you achieving your daily goals and other problem areas.

Yet, the simple truth is inescapable. Eating a varied and nutritious diet together with being more active is the best, most effective and safest way to assure a fit and healthy life for your family – both now and in the future. And you are the one who will have to subtly remind your child of this no-nonsense, it-does-what-it-says-on-the-tin approach to healthy living when the 'magic' solutions grab his attention, as they inevitably will from time to time.

In truth, it is impossible and impractical to try to prevent your child from hearing about these fads. And when they do, you should not deride them too loudly or too soundly. As we've all learned over the years, the fastest way to make something attractive to an adolescent is to ban it.

On the contrary, you should encourage your child to look more closely at the hype surrounding the latest 'exercise craze' or 'fad diet'. It is only in that way that you can discuss the matter with him and help him to make a reasonable judgement about whether or not the new claims have any merits.

You can provide the sensible, non-sensational perspective that will help your child develop and maintain his own realistic approach to fitness and health. Examining these fads and foibles as they surface and calmly discussing their content – with a sense of humour if possible – will help your child see that the claims are usually exaggerated, and many are downright ridiculous – if not dangerous.

Offering support

As your child moves into his secondary education and becomes more independent, so there will be more demands on his free time. Like adults, he will have less and less time to be active – perhaps he has a paper round and, as a result, has had to drop after-school sports clubs. Perhaps the demands of more homework and a busier social life means he is less keen to kick a ball on the field in his rare leisure moments.

Hopefully, if over the years you have instilled in him a love of activity and an understanding of the importance of healthy eating, the message will stay with him and, despite the additional pressures, he will keep the inclination going to be active.

In fact, you may be surprised at the number of adolescents and teens who are keen to maintain fitness and who, completely unprompted, will seize the initiative and go for a run, grab a quick swim or sign up for an exercise class. Interestingly, it is not the dire warnings about future heart attacks that cut any ice with this age group. More often than not, their decision to exercise is influenced by the immediate and tangible effects of being active such as:

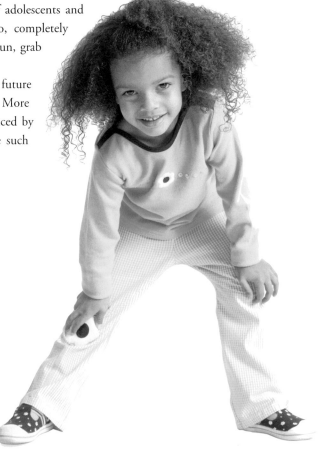

- increased energy

- feelings of well-being

- reduced stress

- firmer and fitter body.

Whatever his reasons for choosing to remain active, you can help him to continue to fit activity into a busy schedule by:

- Being active yourself and including him whenever possible.

- Still offering active family outings and holidays.

- Keeping an eye on the number of hours spent in front of the TV and computer screen.

- Offering to drive him to and from activities if public transport is proving an obstacle.

- Buying home exercise equipment, or paying for club fees/gym membership fees, if possible.

- Offering to be an exercise partner or sport partner for tennis, for example.

- Putting the emphasis on individual sports that he can pursue for a lifetime such as swimming, cycling, hiking, golf or tennis.

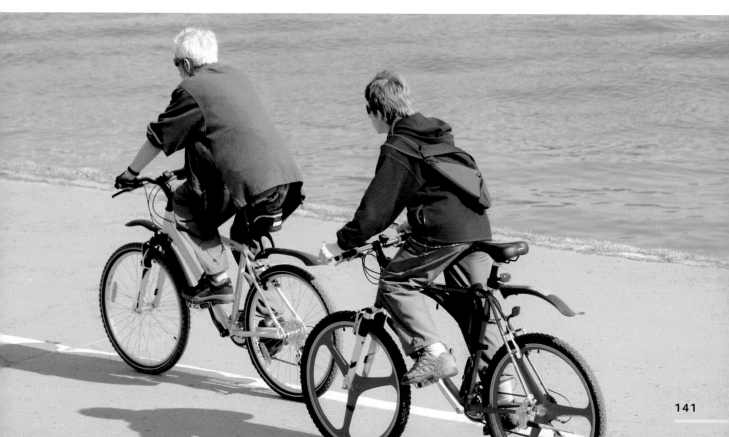

BEWARE THE CONVERT

Like all converts, those who discover the benefits of a more active lifestyle later in life can become the biggest zealots. So, while I hesitate to quash your buoyant enthusiasm, I caution against becoming an exercise fanatic.

As you experience the benefits of being more active, it can be tempting to go to extremes such as banning all TV or insisting on an early morning, pre-breakfast run for the whole family. Don't do it.

Firstly, such extreme measures can backfire spectacularly. If you set yourself up as the one member of the family who becomes conspicuously exasperated by your partner and child's laissez-faire attitude to being active, you are likely to create a 'you vs. them' rift. As you become more and more controlling, so you also become more eccentric and ostracized in the eyes of the rest of your family – and this is definitely counter productive.

Despite your understandable zeal, you are looking for moderation as in all things. So rather than caving in completely on the sofa-hogging or taking the hard line and going for complete bans, look for the middle path where your child is able to watch his favourite programme when you return from a family cycling adventure.

Changes that last a lifetime

We have seen that public health initiatives, miracle diets and exercise remedies may come and go but, ultimately, the key to your family's fitness and good health lies in your hands (and theirs).

The foundation for your child's future health and fitness is laid down and built at home. As you introduce your child to the benefits and pleasures of being more active and eating healthy foods, so you are helping him to achieve lifelong results.

It may be a down-to-earth approach but you may well be

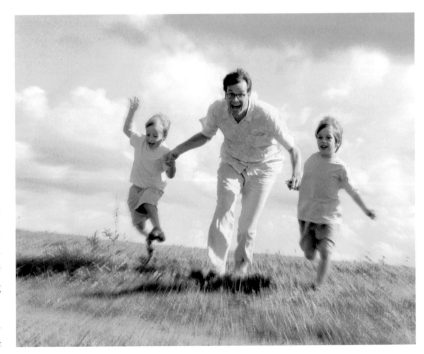

surprised at how positively your family responds to the new lifestyle changes that you are introducing now, and by the many enjoyable 'advantages' that they reap, both as individuals and as a family.

Watching your children being active and doing active pursuits as a family is immensely rewarding and fun. It may take effort to instigate but it soon brings its own rewards and, once experienced, I doubt you will ever want to return to a less active way of life.

Don't expect any thanks for your efforts, but knowing that you're doing the best for your child's future health and fitness will hopefully be appreciation and reward enough.

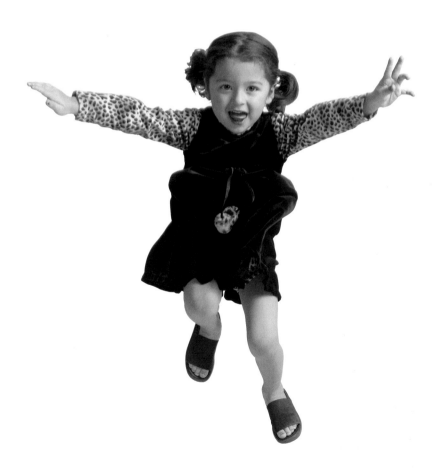

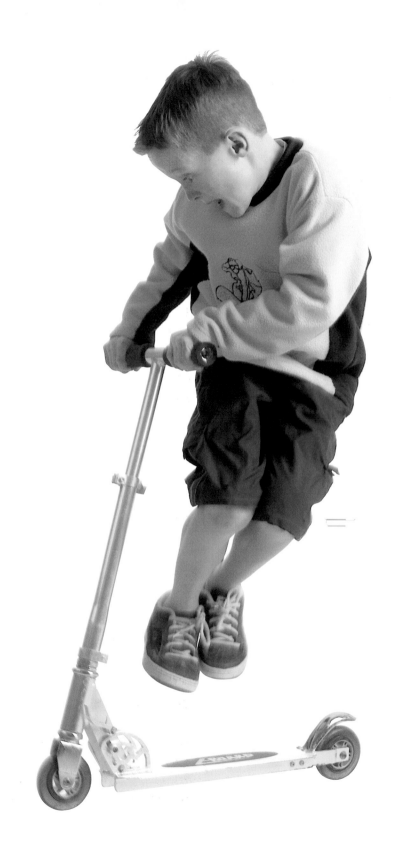

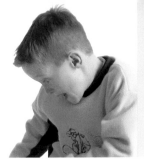

useful contacts

Chapter Two: developing a positive approach

Greatest of All Time (GOAT)

http://www.goatfood.com/

Chapter Three: getting active

British Korfball Association

http://www.korfball.co.uk/

Criminal Records Bureau

www.crb.gov.uk or www.disclosure.gov.uk

Finger Technology

www.fingertech.co.uk

Geocaching

http://www.geocaching.com/

The Guide Association

www.girlguiding.org.uk/

Local Sports Clubs

www.localsportsclubs.co.uk

The Scout Association

www.scoutbase.org.uk

UK Youth Clubs

www.ukyouth.org.uk

YMCA

www.ymcafit.org.uk

Youth Clubs and Groups (Scotland)

www.youthscotland.org.uk

Holiday companies

Club La Manga

Tel: 01869 354100

www.lamangadirect.co.uk

Club La Santa

http://www.clublasanta.com/

Explore Worldwide Ltd

Tel: 01252 760 000

www.explore.co.uk/familyadventures

Mark Warner

Tel: 020 7761 7250

www.markwarner.co.uk

Plas Menai

The National Watersports Centre

Tel: 01248 670964

Brochure Request line: 01248 670597

www.plasmenai.co.uk

Ski Esprit

Tel: 01252 618300

www.esprit-holidays.co.uk

Ski Famille

Tel: 01223 363777.

www.skifamille.co.uk

Chapter Four: getting inspiration

Active Places

Lists sports and fitness facilities anywhere across England

www.activeplaces.com

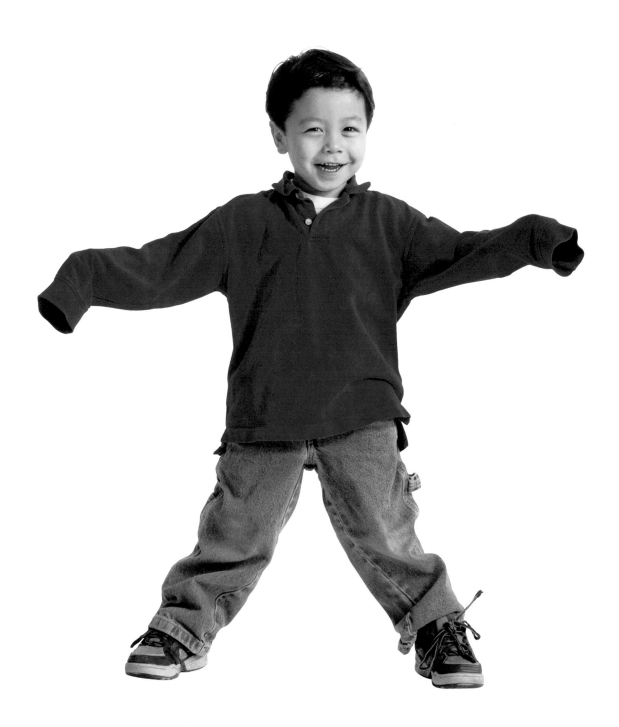

Bobby Charlton Soccer Schools and Sports Academy
http://www.bcssa.co.uk/

British Association of Advisers and Lecturers in Physical Education
www.baalpe.org

The Child Protection in Sport Unit (CPSU)
Website: www.thecpsu.org.uk
Email: cpsu@nspcc.org.uk
Tel: 0116 234 7278

The CPSU (Scotland) Tel: 0141 418 5670
The CPSU (Wales) Tel: 02920 267000

Criminal Records Bureau
www.crb.gov.uk
www.disclosure.gov.uk for information
about the disclosure service
Helpline: 0870 90 90 811

David Beckham Football Academy
http://www.thedavidbeckhamacademy.com/

Department for Culture, Media and Sport
www.dcms.gov.uk/sport

Department for Education and Skills
www.dfes.gov.uk
www.teachernet.gov.uk/pe

Diabetes UK (formerly The British Diabetics Association)
http://www.diabetes.org.uk

The Food Dudes Programme
http://www.fooddudes.co.uk/

Jamie Oliver Feed Me Better Campaign (Campaign to provide real school food)
http://www.feedmebetter.com/

Jamie Oliver School Dinners Campaign
http://www.channel4.com/life/microsites/J/jamies_school_dinners/index.html

Juvenile Diabetes Research Foundation
19 Angel Gate
City Road
London
EC1V 2PT
www.jdrf.org.uk

National Council for School Sport
www.ncss.org.uk

Norwich Union Athletics Sponsorship
www.norwichunion.com/sponsorship

NSPCC
Helpline 0808 800 5000
www.nspcc.org.uk

Physical Education Association of the United Kingdom
www.pea.uk.com

Running Sport
Tel: 0207 404 2224
runningsport@coachwise.ltd.uk

Sportcoach UK
www.sportscoachuk.org
Tel: 01509 226130
Email: bsc@sportscoachuk.org

Sports Council for Wales
www.sports-council-wales.co.uk

Sport England
www.sportengland.org.uk

Sport Scotland
www.sportscotland.org.uk

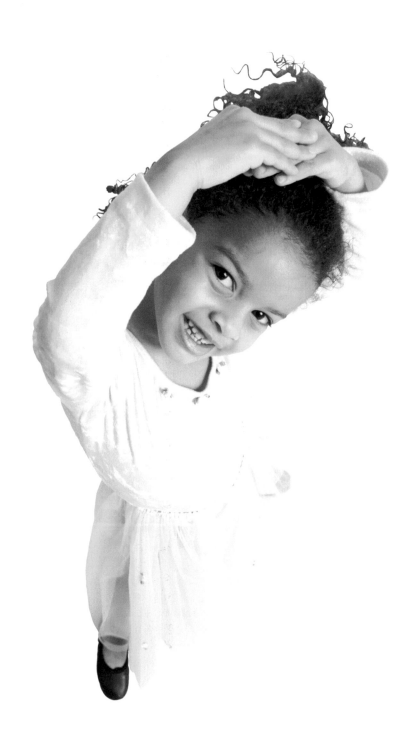

UK Athletics
www.ukathletics.net

Wheelpower (British Wheelchair Sport)
www.wheelpower.org.uk
Tel: 01296 395995

Youth Sport Trust
www.youthsporttrust.org

Chapter Five: good food attitude

The American Dietetic Association
www.eatright.org

The British Nutrition Foundation
www.nutrition.org.uk

Child Growth Foundation
The latest products, information and developments in
child health may be purchased at the shop at
www.healthforallchildren.co.uk

The Food Commission
www.foodcomm.org.uk

Parent Know How
Government campaign suggesting ways in which you can
spend more time together with your child
www.direct.gov.uk/parentknowhow

UK BMI Charts
available from Harlow Printing
www.harlowprinting.co.uk

Chapter Six: activity for big kids

The British Dietetic Association
http://www.bdaweightwise.com

Bullying Online
www.bullying.co.uk

Carnegie Weight Management Camp
Tel: 0113 283 2600 ext: 5233
www.carnegieweightmanagement.com

Childline
Helpline: 0800 1111
www.childline.org.uk

Depression Alliance
020 7633 0557 for a copy of their booklet: The Young
Person's Guide to Stress
www.depressionalliance.org/

Kidscape
Helpline: 08451 205 204
www.kidscape.org.uk

National Obesity Forum
www.nationalobesityforum.org.uk

Parentline Plus
Helpline: 0808 800 222
www.parentlineplus.org.uk

TOAST UK (The Obesity Awareness And Solutions Trust)
www.toast-uk.org

Weight Concern
www.weightconcern.org.uk

YoungMinds Parents Information Service
Tel: 020 7336 8445
www.youngminds.org.uk

Sports national governing bodies

The All England Netball Association Ltd
http://www.englandnetball.co.uk/

The Amateur Rowing Association
http://www.ara-rowing.org/

The Amateur Swimming Association
http://www.britishswimming.org/

The Association of British Riding Schools
Tel: 01736 369440

Badminton England
http://www.badmintonengland.co.uk/

Basketball England
http://www.englandbasketball.co.uk/

The British Canoe Union
http://www.bcu.org.uk/

British Cycling
http://www.britishcycling.org.uk/development/Clubs_intro.html

British Gymnastics
http://www.british-gymnastics.org/

The British Horse Society (Horse riding)
www.bhs.org.uk

British Judo
http://www.britishjudo.org.uk/

The British Orienteering Federation
http://www.britishorienteering.org.uk/

British Surfing Association
www.britsurf.co.uk

Children In Golf
http://www.childreningolf.co.uk/

The England and Wales Cricket Board
http://www.ecb.co.uk/safehands

England Hockey
http://www.hockeyonline.co.uk/

England Squash
http://www.englandsquash.com/

The England Table Tennis Association
http://www.englishtabletennis.org.uk/

The English Volleyball Association
http://www.volleyballengland.org/

The Football Association
http://www.thefa.com/

In-line Skating Instructors
www.icp-international.org

The Lawn Tennis Association
http://www.lta.org.uk/

The Royal Yachting Association
http://www.rya.org.uk/

The Rugby Football League
http://www.rfl.uk.com/

The Rugby Football Union
http://www.rfu.com/

UK Athletics
http://www.ukathletics.net/

index